Series Editor: S

MW00652276

Stahl's Neuroscience
and Mental Health
Pocketbook Series

Antipsychotics

Stephen M. Stahl
University of California at San Diego

Nancy Muntner
Illustrations

Laurence Mignon
Editor

NEI Press
www.neiglobal.com

Every effort has been made in preparing this book to provide accurate and up-to-date information that is in accord with accepted standards and practice at the time of publication. Nevertheless, the author, editors, and publisher can make no warranties that the information contained herein is totally free from error, not least because clinical standards are constantly changing through research and regulation. The author, editors, and publisher therefore disclaim all liability for direct or consequential damages resulting from the use of material contained in this book. Readers are strongly advised to pay careful attention to information provided by the manufacturer of any drugs or equipment that they plan to use.

PUBLISHED BY NEI PRESS, an imprint of
NEUROSCIENCE EDUCATION INSTITUTE
Carlsbad, California, United States of America

NEUROSCIENCE EDUCATION INSTITUTE
1930 Palomar Point Way, Suite 101
Carlsbad, California 92008

http://www.neiglobal.com

Copyright © 2008 Neuroscience Education Institute.
All rights reserved.

This publication is in copyright. Subject to statutory exception and to the provisions of relevant collective licensing agreements, no reproduction of any part may take place without the written permission of Neuroscience Education Institute.

Printed in the United States of America
First Edition, April 2008

Typeset in Futura

Library of Congress Cataloging-in-Publication Data
ISBN 1-4225-0046-2

PREFACE

These books are designed to be fun. All concepts are illustrated by full-color images. The text can be used as a supplement to figures, images, and tables. The visual learner will find that this book makes psychopharmacology concepts easy to master, while the non-visual learner may enjoy a shortened text version of complex psychopharmacology concepts. Each chapter builds upon previous chapters, synthesizing information from basic biology and diagnostics to building treatment plans and dealing with complications and comorbidities.

Novices may want to approach this Pocketbook by first looking through all the graphics, gaining a feel for the visual vocabulary on which our psychopharmacology concepts rely. After this once-over glance, we suggest going back through the book to incorporate the images with text from figure legends. Learning from visual concepts and textual supplements should reinforce one another, providing you with solid conceptual understanding at each step along the way.

Readers more familiar with these topics should find that going back and forth between images and text provides an interaction with which to vividly conceptualize complex psychopharmacology. You may find yourself using this book frequently to refresh your psychopharmacological knowledge. And you will hopefully refer your colleagues to this desk reference.

This Pocketbook is intended as a conceptual overview of different topics; we provide you with a visual-based language to incorporate the rules of psychopharmacology at the sacrifice of discussing the exceptions to these rules. A Suggested Readings section at the end of this Pocketbook gives you a good start for more in-depth learning about particular concepts presented here.

When you come across an abbreviation or figure you don't understand, you can refer to the Abbreviation and Symbols legend in the back. After referring to these several times you will begin to develop proficiency in the visual vocabulary of psychopharmacology. Stahl's Essential Psychopharmacology, 3rd Edition, and Stahl's Essential Psychopharmacology: The Prescriber's Guide, 2nd Edition, can be helpful supplementary tools for more in-depth information on particular topics in this Pocketbook. Now you can also search topics in psychopharmacology on the Neuroscience Education Institute's website (www.neiglobal.com) for lectures, courses, slides and related articles.

Whether you are a novice or an experienced psychopharmacologist, hopefully this book will lead you to think critically about the complexities involved in psychiatric disorders and their treatments.

Best wishes for your educational journey into the fascinating field of psychopharmacology!

Stephen M. Stahl

Table of Contents

CME Information

Overview
This book aims to visually explain the underlying pathophysiology of schizophrenia, give an overview of the receptor profiles of conventional and atypical antipsychotics and provide information on best treatment approaches. The book is divided into five chapters for ease of reading and referencing. Chapter 1 <u>Neurobiology of Schizophrenia</u> focuses on the known and hypothetical causes underlying the pathophysiology of schizophrenia. Chapter 2 <u>Three Classes of Antipsychotics</u> is divided into three parts and focuses on conventional D2 antagonists, 5HT2A/D2 antagonists, and D2 partial agonists. Chapter 3 <u>Side Effects of Antipsychotics: Metabolic Issues and Sedation</u> explains the importance of monitoring patients initiated on antipsychotic medication. Chapter 4 <u>Seventeen Antipsychotic Drugs</u> describes each antipsychotic medication currently available in terms of side effects profile, dosing tips, and drug interactions. Finally, Chapter 5 <u>Schizophrenia Pharmacy and Switching Strategies</u> presents different ways to treat the various symptoms of schizophrenia and describes ways to switch between different antipsychotic agents. The visual component of this minibook is designed to allow the reader to easily grasp concepts.

Target Audience
This activity was designed for healthcare professionals, including psychiatrists, neurologists, primary care physicians, nurses, pharmacists, and others who treat patients with psychiatric conditions.

Statement of Need
The following unmet needs regarding antipsychotics were revealed following a vigorous assessment of activity feedback, expert faculty assessment, literature review, and through new medical knowledge:

- The neurobiology underlying schizophrenia is based on the dopamine hypothesis, but many other neurotransmitter systems are also involved. It is important to understand the interaction among these neurotransmitter systems in order to get the full picture of the underlying causes of schizophrenia

- The pharmacological agents used to treat schizophrenia affect neurobiological systems in specific ways; understanding the relationship between the medications and the underlying pathophysiology of schizophrenia is essential in order to select appropriate treatment for a patient

- Acquiring a better knowledge of the different antipsychotics on the market and in development is necessary to ascertain proper dosing and switching strategies and thus to maximize treatment benefits and minimize side effects

- Based on evaluations obtained at NEI Academies, participants wanted more information on psychosis-related matters, and additional information on dosing issues

To help fill these unmeet needs, quality improvement efforts need to increase understanding of the neurobiology of psychiatric disease states and the pharmacology of available, new, and in-development medications.

Learning Objectives

After completing this activity, participants should be better able to:

- Describe the hypothetical neurobiology of schizophrenia
- Understand the complex pharmacology of antipsychotics
- Recognize how different drug properties affect the various symptoms of schizophrenia
- Recognize that side effects are linked to the drug's receptor profile
- Develop an understanding of the best treatment practices and switching methods for schizophrenia

Accreditation and Credit Designation Statements

The Neuroscience Education Institute is accredited by the Accreditation Council for Continuing Medical Education to provide continuing medical education for physicians.

The Neuroscience Education Institute designates this educational activity for a maximum of 3.0 *AMA PRA Category 1 Credits*™. Physicians should only claim credit commensurate with the extent of their participation in the activity. Non-physicians may receive a certificate of participation for completing this activity.

Activity Instructions

This CME activity is in the form of a printed monograph and incorporates instructional design to enhance your retention of the information and pharmacological concepts that are being presented. You are advised to go through the figures in this activity from beginning to end, followed by the text, and then complete the posttest and activity evaluation. The estimated time for completion of this activity is 3.0 hours.

Instructions for CME Credit

To receive your certificate of CME credit or participation, please complete the posttest (you must score at least 70% to receive credit) and activity evaluation found at the end of the monograph and mail or fax them to the address/number provided. Once received, your posttest will be graded and a certificate sent if a score of 70% or more was attained. Alternatively, **you may complete the posttest and activity evaluation online and immediately print your certificate**. There is a fee for CME credits for this activity.

NEI Disclosure Policy

It is the policy of the Neuroscience Education Institute to ensure balance, independence, objectivity, and scientific rigor in all its educational activities. Therefore, all individuals in a position to influence or control content development are required by NEI to disclose any financial relationships or apparent conflicts of interest that may have a direct bearing on the subject matter of the activity. Although potential conflicts of interest are identified and resolved prior to the activity being presented, it remains for the participant to determine whether outside interests reflect a possible bias in either the exposition or the conclusions presented.

These materials have been peer-reviewed to ensure the scientific accuracy and medical relevance of information presented and its independence from commercial bias. The Neuroscience Education Institute takes responsibility for the content, quality, and scientific integrity of this CME activity.

Individual Disclosure Statements
Author
Stephen M. Stahl, MD, PhD

Adjunct Professor, Department of Psychiatry, University of California, San Diego School of Medicine

Board Member: Cypress Bioscience, Inc.; NeuroMolecular Pharmaceuticals; Pierre Fabre; Tetragenix Pharmaceuticals

Grant/Research: Alkermes, Inc.; AstraZeneca Pharmaceuticals LP; Bristol-Myers Squibb Company; Cephalon, Inc.; Cyberonics; Eli Lilly and Company; GlaxoSmith-Kline; Janssen Pharmaceutica Inc.; Jazz Pharmaceuticals; Neurocrine Biosciences Inc.; Novartis; Organon; Pfizer Inc; Sepracor Inc.; Shire Pharmaceuticals Inc.; Somaxon Pharmaceuticals, Inc.; Takeda Pharmaceuticals North America, Inc.; Wyeth Pharmaceuticals

Consultant/Advisor: ACADIA Pharmaceuticals Inc.; Amylin Pharmaceuticals, Inc; AstraZeneca Pharmaceuticals LP; Avera Pharmaceuticals, Inc.; Azur Pharma Inc; Biovail Pharmaceuticals, Inc.; Boehringer Ingelheim Pharmaceuticals, Inc.; Bristol-Myers Squibb Company; Cephalon, Inc.; CSC Pharmaceuticals; Cyberonics; Cypress Bioscience, Inc.; Dainippon Pharmaceutical USA Corporation; Eli Lilly and Company; EPIX Pharmaceuticals, Inc.; Forest Pharmaceuticals, Inc.; GlaxoSmithKline; Janssen Pharmaceutica Inc.; Jazz Pharmaceuticals, Inc.; Labopharm Inc.; Neurocrine Biosciences Inc.; NeuroMolecular Pharmaceuticals; Neuronetics, Inc.; Novartis; Organon; Pamlab, L.L.C.; Pfizer Inc; Pierre Fabre; sanofi-aventis U.S. LLC; Schering-Plough Corporation; Sepracor Inc.; Shire Pharmaceuticals Inc.; SK Corporation; Solvay Pharmaceuticals; Somaxon Pharmaceuticals, Inc.; Tethys Pharmaceutical, Inc.; Tetragenix Pharmaceuticals; Vanda Pharmaceuticals Inc.; Wyeth Pharmaceuticals

Speakers Bureau: AstraZeneca Pharmaceuticals LP; Cephalon, Inc.; CSC Pharmaceuticals; Eli Lilly and Company; Pfizer Inc; Wyeth Pharmaceuticals

Content Editors
Laurence Mignon, PhD
Medical Writer, Neuroscience Education Institute, Carlsbad, CA
Stockholder: Aspreva Pharmaceuticals Corporation; Vanda Pharmaceuticals Inc.; ViroPharma Incorporated

Meghan Grady
Director, Content Development, Neuroscience Education Institute, Carlsbad, CA
No other financial relationships to disclose.

Peer Reviewer
Electa Stern, PharmD, CACP
Clinical Supervisor, Pharmacy Services, Sharp Grossmont Hospital, La Mesa, CA
Attended Advisory Board re anti-infective: Johnson & Johnson Pharmaceutical Services, L.L.C.; Pfizer Inc

Design Staff
Nancy Muntner
Director, Medical Illustrations, Neuroscience Education Institute, Carlsbad, CA
No other financial relationships to disclose.

Disclosed financial relationships have been reviewed by the Neuroscience Education Institute CME Advisory Board to resolve any potential conflicts of interest. All faculty and planning committee members have attested that their financial relationships do not affect their ability to present well-balanced, evidence-based content for this activity.

Disclosure of Off-Label Use
This educational activity may include discussion of products or devices that are not currently labeled for such use by the Food and Drug Administration. Please consult the product prescribing information for full disclosure of labeled uses.

Disclaimer
The information presented in this educational activity is not meant to define a standard of care, nor is it intended to dictate an exclusive course of patient management. Any procedures, medications, or other courses of diagnosis or treatment discussed or suggested in this educational activity should not be used by clinicians without full evaluation of their patients' conditions and possible contraindications or dangers in use, review of any applicable manufacturer's product information, and comparison with recommendations of other authorities. Primary references and full prescribing information should be consulted.

Participants have an implied responsibility to use the newly acquired information from this activity to enhance patient outcomes and their own professional development. The participant should use his/her clinical judgment, knowledge, experience, and diagnostic decision-making before applying any information, whether provided here or by others, for any professional use.

Sponsorship Information
This activity is sponsored by Neuroscience Education Institute.

Support
This activity is supported solely by the sponsor, Neuroscience Education Institute. Neither the Neuroscience Education Institute nor Stephen M. Stahl, MD, PhD has received any funds or grants in support of this educational activity.

Date of Release/Expiration
Release Date: May, 2008   CME Credit Expiration Date: April, 2011

Stahl's Neuroscience
and Mental Health
Pocketbook Series | # Objectives

- Describe the hypothetical neurobiology of schizophrenia

- Understand the complex pharmacology of antipsychotics

- Recognize how different drug properties affect the various symptoms of schizo-phrenia

- Recognize that side effects are linked to the drug's receptor profile

- Develop an understanding of the best treatment practices and switching methods for schizophrenia

Chapter 1

Neurobiology of Schizophrenia

This chapter will introduce the neurobiology that is thought to underlie the symptoms of schizophrenia. The dopamine hypothesis of schizophrenia has been accepted for a long time, especially as the first antipsychotics were shown to block dopamine D2 receptors. This theory posits that dopamine is overactive in some brain areas, and underactive in other brain areas. This chapter shows that it might be more accurate to say that dopamine is neither "too high" nor "too low" but "out of tune." In addition, ideas about the involvement of glutamate and serotonin have gained momentum in the pathophysiology of schizophrenia, and this chapter aims to give an overview of how these three neurotransmitter systems may come together to induce both the positive and negative symptoms of schizophrenia. This brief overview will also aid in understanding the occurrence of side effects of different antipsychotics.

Antipsychotics Overview

Class	Name
Conventional APs	Chlorpromazine, cyamemazine, fluphenthixol, fluphenazine, haloperidol, loxapine, mesoridazine, molindone, perphenazine, pimozide, pipothiazine, sulpiride, thioridazine, thiothixene, trifluoperazine, zuclopenthixol
SDAs	Clozapine, risperidone, paliperidone, olanzapine, quetiapine, ziprasidone, perospirone, zotepine, sertindole, low-dose loxapine?, low-dose cyamemazine?
SDAs in development	Iloperidone, asenapine, SM13493/lurasidone, blonanserin, Y931, NRA0562, nemonapride
DPAs	Aripiprazole, low-dose sulpiride?, amisulpride?
DPAs in development	Bifeprunox, sarizotan, RGH188, 3PPP, SLV313, SLV314, ACR16, PNU 9639/OSU 6162, CI1007, ACP-104, SSR-181507
SPAs	SPA + SDA: ziprasidone, quetiapine, clozapine SDA + DPA + SPA: aripiprazole DPA + SPA: bifeprunox

AP: antipsychotic; SDA: serotonin 2A dopamine 2 antagonist; DPA: dopamine 2 partial agonist; SPA: serotonin 1A partial agonist

TABLE 1.1. Since the discovery of chlorpromazine in the 1950s, the development of new antipsychotics has been based mainly on their ability to block dopamine 2 receptors. Additional properties have been integrated into the newer medications to improve therapeutic efficacy and prevent/reduce drug-related side effects. This table provides an overview of the different types of antipsychotics used to date.

Key Brain Regions and Their Hypothetical Functions

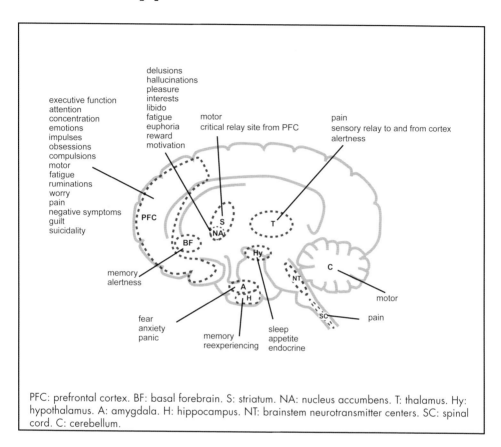

PFC: prefrontal cortex. BF: basal forebrain. S: striatum. NA: nucleus accumbens. T: thalamus. Hy: hypothalamus. A: amygdala. H: hippocampus. NT: brainstem neurotransmitter centers. SC: spinal cord. C: cerebellum.

FIGURE 1.1. Psychiatric disorders hypothetically result from alterations in neurotransmission within different brain regions. A different set of symptoms is unveiled depending on which brain area is functionally impaired.

In schizophrenia, the neurotransmitter dopamine (DA) is theoretically dysregulated, and as a result various brain areas are overactive, underactive, or otherwise "out of tune," resulting in the generation of positive and negative symptoms.

Key DA Pathways

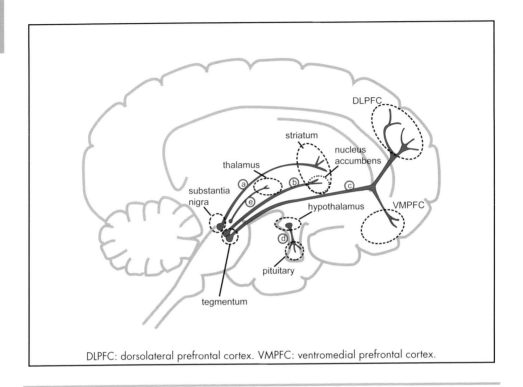

DLPFC: dorsolateral prefrontal cortex. VMPFC: ventromedial prefrontal cortex.

FIGURE 1.2. Five dopamine (DA) pathways are relevant in explaining the symptoms of schizophrenia and the therapeutic and side effects of antipsychotic drugs.

(a) The nigrostriatal DA pathway is part of the extrapyramidal nervous system, which controls motor function and movement.

(b) The mesolimbic DA pathway is part of the brain's limbic system, which regulates behaviors including pleasurable sensations, the powerful euphoria of drugs of abuse, and the delusions and hallucinations seen in psychosis.

(c) The mesocortical DA pathway is implicated in mediating the cognitive symptoms (dorsolateral prefrontal cortex, DLPFC) and affective symptoms (ventromedial prefrontal cortex, VMPFC) of schizophrenia.

(d) The tuberoinfundibular DA pathway projects from the hypothalamus to the anterior pituitary gland and controls prolactin secretion.

(e) The fifth DA pathway arises from multiple sites, including the periaqueductal gray, ventral mesencephalon, hypothalamic nuclei, and lateral parabrachial nucleus and projects to the thalamus. Its function is not well known.

The DA Hypothesis of Schizophrenia: Positive Symptoms

MESOLIMBIC DOPAMINE PATHWAY

normal

HIGH

overactivation
normal
baseline
hypoactivation

mesolimbic overactivity = positive symptoms of schizophrenia

positive symptoms

FIGURE 1.3. The mesolimbic DA pathway sends DA projections from cell bodies in the ventral tegmental area to the nucleus accumbens in the ventral striatum. This pathway hypothetically regulates emotional behaviors, pleasure, and reward and is the main candidate thought to regulate the positive symptoms of psychosis. Specifically, it has been hypothesized that hyperactivity of this pathway accounts for the delusions and hallucinations observed in schizophrenia. This hypothesis is known both as the "DA hypothesis of schizophrenia" and perhaps more precisely as the "mesolimbic DA hyperactivity hypothesis of positive symptoms of schizophrenia."

The DA Hypothesis of Schizophrenia:
Negative, Cognitive, and Affective Symptoms

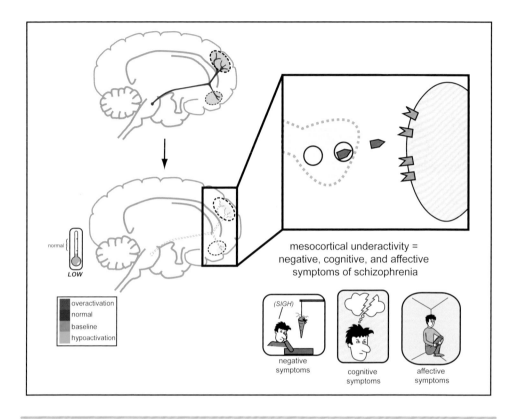

mesocortical underactivity =
negative, cognitive, and affective
symptoms of schizophrenia

normal
LOW

overactivation
normal
baseline
hypoactivation

(SIGH)

negative
symptoms

cognitive
symptoms

affective
symptoms

FIGURE 1.4. The mesocortical DA pathway is hypothetically also affected in schizophrenia. Here, DA cell bodies in the ventral tegmental area send projections to the DLPFC to regulate cognition and executive functions, and to the VMPFC to regulate emotions and affect. Hypoactivation of this pathway theoretically results in the negative, cognitive, and affective symptoms seen in schizophrenia. This hypothesis is sometimes called the "mesocortical DA hypothesis of negative, cognitive, and affective symptoms" of schizophrenia. This DA deficit could result from ongoing degeneration due to glutamate excitotoxicity or from a neurodevelopmental impairment in the glutamatergic system.

Loss of motivation and interest, anhedonia, and lack of pleasure as observed in schizophrenia result not only from a malfunctioning mesocortical DA pathway but also from a deficient mesolimbic DA pathway.

Additional DA Pathways

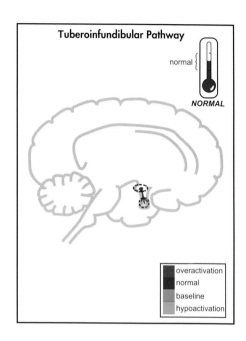

FIGURE 1.5. The nigrostriatal pathway sends DA projections from the substantia nigra to the striatum. This innervation of the basal ganglia regulates motor activity and is part of the extrapyramidal nervous system. A lack of DA here results in symptoms resembling Parkinson's disease, whereas an excess of DA will lead to hyperkinetic movement disorders such as dyskinesias.

FIGURE 1.6. DA inhibits prolactin secretion via the tuberoinfundibular pathway as DA projections are sent from the hypothalamus to the anterior pituitary.

Although these two pathways are unaffected in schizophrenia, they do play an intricate part in the development of side effects, as they will not remain untouched by drugs interacting with DA neurons throughout the brain.

The Integrated DA Hypothesis of Schizophrenia

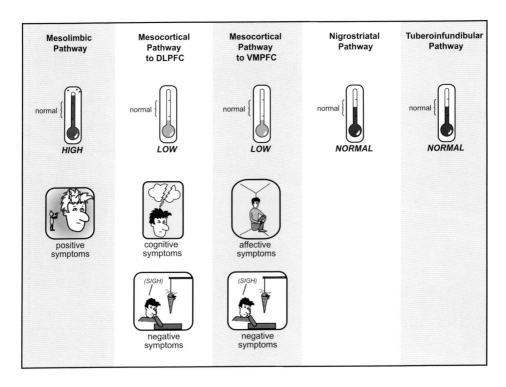

FIGURE 1.7. In schizophrenia, it appears that some DA pathways are overactive, others underactive and others are functioning normally. Thus the DA system is neither "all too high" nor "all too low" but more precisely "out of tune," and DA needs to be increased in some areas, decreased in others and left untouched in yet another set of circuits.

Various antipsychotic drugs acting at different receptor subtypes, especially blocking D2 receptors and serotonin 2A (5HT2A) receptors, might lead to that outcome.

Alternatively, regulating DA output by modulating transmitters such as glutamate may prove to be another way to "normalize" or "tune" DA circuits.

Key Glutamate Pathways

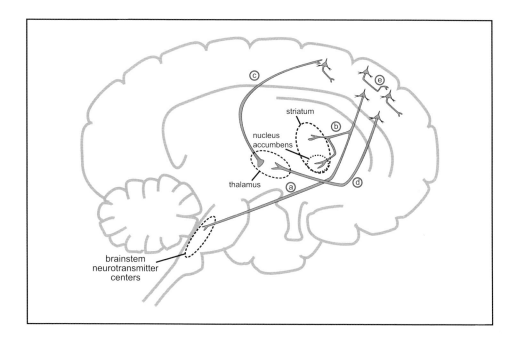

FIGURE 1.8. Similarly to DA, there are five glutamate pathways in the brain that are of particular relevance to schizophrenia.

(a) The <u>cortical brainstem glutamate projection</u> descends from layer 5 pyramidal neurons in the prefrontal cortex (PFC) to brainstem neurotransmitter centers, including the raphe (5HT), the locus coeruleus (norepinephrine) and the ventral tegmental area and substantia nigra (DA). This projection mainly regulates neurotransmitter release in the brainstem.

(b) The <u>cortico-striatal glutamate pathway</u> descends from the PFC to the striatum and the <u>cortico-accumbens glutamate pathway</u> sends projections to the nucleus accumbens. These pathways make up the "cortico-striatal" portion of cortico-striatal-thalamic loops.

(c) <u>Thalamo-cortical glutamate pathways</u> encompass pathways ascending from the thalamus and innervating pyramidal neurons in the cortex.

(d) <u>Cortico-thalamic glutamate pathways</u> descend from the PFC to the thalamus.

(e) The <u>cortico-cortical glutamatergic pathways</u> allow intracortical pyramidal neurons to communicate with each other.

NMDA Receptor Hypofunction Hypothesis of Schizophrenia

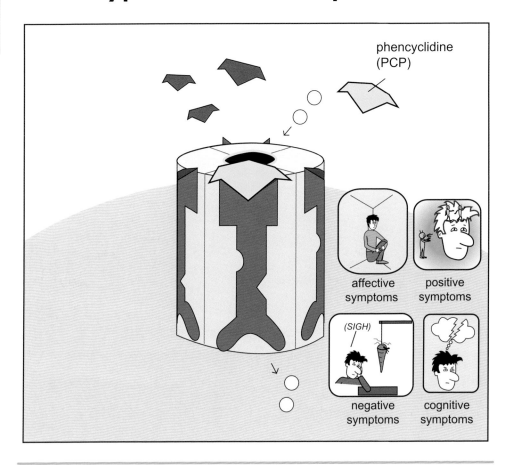

FIGURE 1.9. The NMDA (N-methyl-d-aspartate) receptor hypofunction hypothesis has been put forth in an attempt to explain mesolimbic DA hyperactivity. This hypothesis relies on the observation that when normal humans ingest phencyclidine (PCP), an NMDA receptor antagonist, they experience positive symptoms very similar to those observed in schizophrenia such as hallucinations and delusions. Thus hypoactive glutamate NMDA receptors could theoretically explain the biological basis for the mesolimbic DA hyperactivity. PCP also induces affective symptoms such as blunted affect, negative symptoms such as social withdrawal, and cognitive symptoms such as executive dysfunction in normal humans. Hypofunctional NMDA receptors might therefore be involved in all symptoms of schizophrenia.

Role of Glutamate in the Mesolimbic System

How might glutamatergic and dopaminergic pathways in the mesolimbic system lead to positive symptoms in schizophrenia?

normal

HIGH

DA neuron

GLU neuron

GABA neuron

A

B

positive symptoms

- overactivation
- normal
- baseline
- hypoactivation

FIGURE 1.10. Various theories have been put forth trying to explain the overactivity of the DA pathway in the mesolimbic system in schizophrenia. The descending cortico-brainstem glutamate pathway normally acts as a brake for the mesolimbic DA pathway, via gamma-aminobutyric acid (GABA) interneurons in the ventral tegmental area, leading to a tonic inhibition of the mesolimbic DA pathway (A).

If glutamate projections become hypoactive, this tonic inhibition of the mesolimbic DA pathway will not occur, leading to hyperactivity in the mesolimbic DA pathway (B).

Role of Glutamate in the Mesocortical System

How might glutamatergic pathways in the mesocortical system lead to negative symptoms in schizophrenia?

FIGURE 1.11. Normally, the cortico-brainstem glutamate projections synapse directly onto DA neurons in the ventral tegmental area, where they tonically excite the mesocortical DA pathway and act as DA neuron accelerators (A).

Hypoactivity in glutamate projections, similarly to what is observed following PCP administration, can thus theoretically result in lost activation of the mesocortical DA neurons and might be the cause of the negative, cognitive, and affective symptoms seen in schizophrenia (B).

Key Serotonin Pathways

PFC: prefrontal cortex. BF: basal forebrain. S: striatum. NA: nucleus accumbens. T: thalamus. Hy: hypothalamus. A: amygdala. H: hippocampus. NT: brainstem neurotransmitter centers. SC: spinal cord. C: cerebellum.

FIGURE 1.12. In order to fully understand the properties of antipsychotics, it is imperative to examine the serotonin (5HT) pathways throughout the brain and how they modulate DA and glutamate circuits.

Ascending 5HT projections originate in the raphe nucleus in the brainstem and extend to many of the same regions as noradrenergic projections, with additional projections to the striatum and nucleus accumbens. These ascending projections may regulate mood, anxiety, sleep, and other functions. Descending 5HT projections extend down the brainstem and through the spinal cord and may regulate pain.

Opposing Actions of 5HT1A and 5HT2A Receptors on DA Release

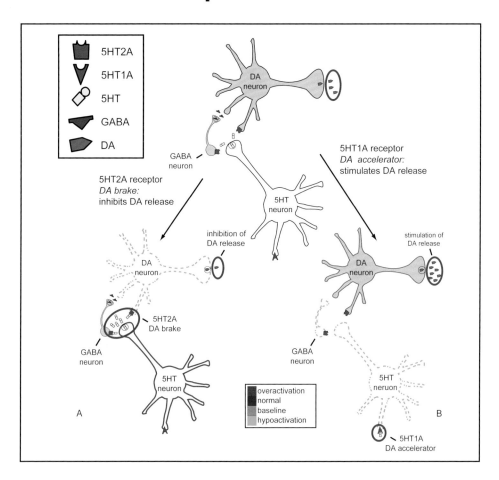

FIGURE 1.13. 5HT neurons can act on somatodendritic regions of DA neurons. Specifically, 5HT1A and 5HT2A receptors have opposite actions on DA release. Stimulation of 5HT1A receptors increases DA release, and thus 5HT1A receptors act as a DA accelerator. Stimulation of 5HT2A receptors inhibits DA release; thus 5HT2A receptors act as a DA brake. 5HT can regulate DA release directly or indirectly. (A) When 5HT binds to 5HT2A receptors on DA neurons or on GABA neurons, DA release is decreased directly or via inhibition through GABA release, respectively. (B) Upon binding to 5HT1A receptors, 5HT causes inhibition of its own release. A lack of 5HT results in disinhibition of DA release, and therefore increased DA output.

Somatodendritic Blockade of 5HT2A Receptors Leads to Increased DA Release

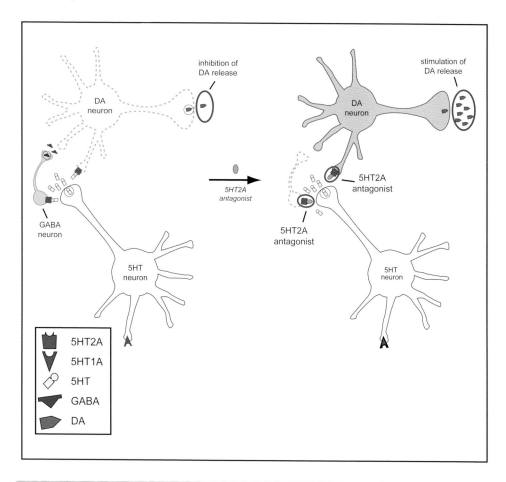

FIGURE 1.14. If stimulation of 5HT2A receptors leads to decreased DA release, then blocking 5HT2A receptors via antagonists should result in increased DA release. Increasing DA release can therefore be obtained by either blocking 5HT2A receptors on postsynaptic DA neurons or by blocking 5HT2A receptors on GABA interneurons.

Regulation of DA Release by 5HT in the Nigrostriatal Pathway: Part 1

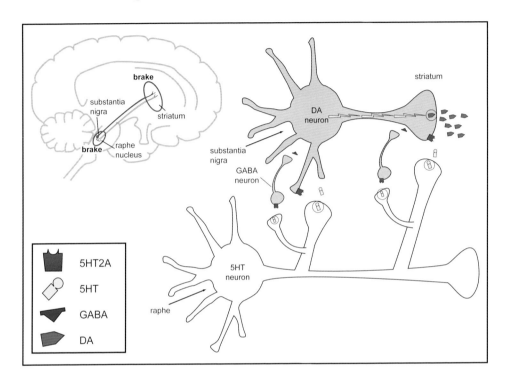

FIGURE 1.15. The 5HT-DA interaction at the level of the nigrostriatal pathway is important in mediating extrapyramidal side effects. Here 5HT can regulate DA release by acting on the somatodendritic regions of the DA neuron in the substantia nigra, or by acting on the axonal regions of the DA neuron in the striatum.

Part 1: In the absence of 5HT, DA is freely released in the striatum.

Regulation of DA Release by 5HT in the Nigrostriatal Pathway: Part 2

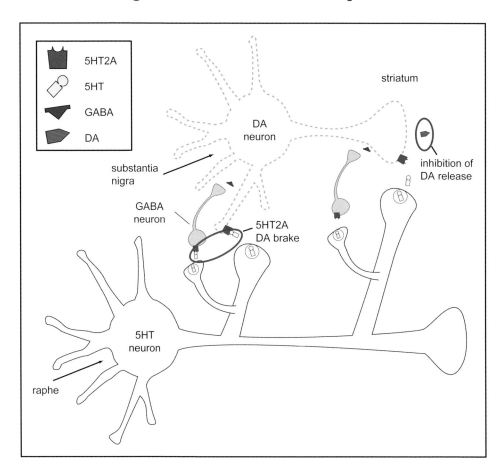

FIGURE 1.16. Part 2: When 5HT is released from raphe projections to the substantia nigra (red circle on the left), it will stimulate postsynaptic somatodendritic 5HT2A receptors on DA and GABA neurons. This will lead to inhibition of axonal DA release (red circle on the right).

Regulation of DA Release by 5HT in the Nigrostriatal Pathway: Part 3

FIGURE 1.17. Part 3: When 5HT is released from a synaptic connection projecting from axoaxonal contacts or by volume neurotransmission between 5HT and DA axon terminals (red circle, bottom), it will stimulate postsynaptic 5HT2A receptors on DA and GABA neurons, leading to decreased axonal DA release (red circle, top).

What Happens at the Axon Terminal in the Striatum?

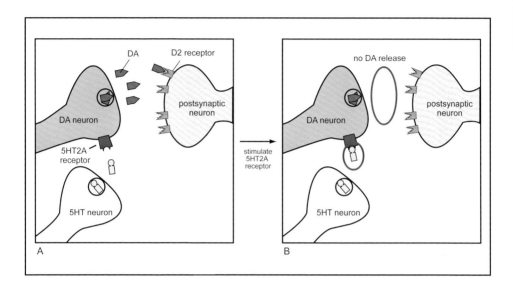

FIGURE 1.18. At the level of striatal axons, 5HT normally inhibits DA release. (A) In the absence of 5HT, however, DA is released without hindrance. (B) In the presence of 5HT, 5HT2A receptors on DA terminals are stimulated, thus inhibiting DA release, thereby leading to a lack of synaptic DA.

5HT Also Modulates Cortical Glutamate Release

FIGURE 1.19. Stimulation of 5HT2A and 5HT1A receptors also leads to an opposing modulation of cortical glutamate release, but does so contrary to the actions of these same 5HT receptors upon DA release. Here, stimulation of 5HT2A receptors located on glutamate cell bodies induces an increase in glutamate release, acting as a glutamate accelerator.

Stimulation of 5HT1A receptors located on glutamate axons inhibits glutamate release, acting as a glutamate brake.

As already mentioned, this is contrary to the regulation that 5HT has on DA release (see Figs. 1.15-18), where stimulation of 5HT1A receptors leads to increased DA release (accelerator) and stimulation of 5HT2A receptors leads to inhibition of DA release (brake).

Strengthening the Signal-to-Noise Ratio in Schizophrenia

| signals from multiple inputs to cortical pyramidal neurons | neurotransmitter input can "tune" cortical pyramidal neurons by increasing the signal and decreasing the noise (enhancing signal-to-noise ratio) | cortical pyramidal neurons and neurotransmitters: more is not always better |

multiple competing signals   *"tuning" enhances signal-to-noise ratio*   receptor stimulation / pyramidal neuronal functioning

A   B   C

FIGURE 1.20. (A) Adequate information processing occurs when all neurotransmitters are working in tune. In schizophrenia, however, information processing in specific key brain areas is abnormal.

Prefrontal cortical activity in schizophrenia is not just "too high" or "too low," but it is most likely "out of tune" or "chaotic," with some areas hyperactive and others hypoactive.

(B) When prefrontal neurons are adequately tuned, the signal-to-noise ratio is sensitive enough to allow for proper filtering of "noise," resulting in the strengthening of one signal over another.

(C) As represented by the inverted U-shaped curve, moderation is preferable when it comes to receptor stimulation. Too much or too little stimulation is suboptimal. Thus in order to reach the optimal tuning of the signal-to-noise ratio it is important to determine where the system is on the curve, as it might need to be either increased or decreased.

Chapter 2

Three Classes of Antipsychotics

The serendipitous discovery in the 1950s that the antihistamine chlorpromazine can relieve symptoms of psychosis led to the discovery of conventional antipsychotics. Their ability to block D2 receptors was recognized by the 1970s. Since then, much research has been done to improve antipsychotic medications. This chapter covers three topics: exploring the different classes of antipsychotics, explaining their mechanisms of action, and describing how they affect the brain circuitry introduced in Chapter 1.

Section 1: Conventional D2 Antagonists
Section 2: Atypical 5HT2A/D2 Antagonists
Section 3: D2 Partial Agonists

– SECTION 1 –
Conventional D2 Antagonists

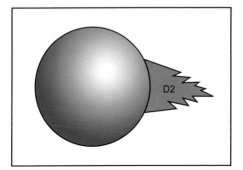

FIGURE 2.1. Conventional antipsychotics treat the symptoms of schizophrenia by blocking D2 receptors. Excessive blockade of D2 receptors, or blockade of DA receptors in hypoactive areas can lead to many side effects, including "neurolepsis," an extreme form of slowness or absence of motor movement, as well as the worsening of negative, cognitive, and affective symptoms.

Conventional Antipsychotics	
Generic Name	**Trade Name**
Chlorpromazine	Thorazine
Cyamemazine	Terican
Fluphenthixol	Depixol
Fluphenazine	Prolixin
Haloperidol	Haldol
Loxapine	Loxitane
Mesoridazine	Serentil
Molindone	Moban
Perphenazine	Trilafon
Pimozide	Orap
Pipothiazine	Piportil
Sulpiride	Dolmatil
Thioridazine	Mellaril
Thiothixene	Navane
Trifluoperazine	Stelazine
Zuclopenthixol	Clopixol

TABLE 2.1. Some of the conventional antipsychotics in use today.

D2 Antagonism in the Mesolimbic DA Pathway

FIGURE 2.2. As excess DA release in the mesolimbic DA pathway leads to positive symptoms, it is necessary to reduce the actions of DA here in order to normalize the situation. Administration of a D2 blocker, such as any conventional antipsychotic, prevents DA from binding to the D2 receptor.

This D2 antagonism will lead to a reduction in both the hyperactivity of this pathway and the positive symptoms linked to it.

However, the mesolimbic DA pathway is not the only pathway affected by D2 antagonists.

D2 Antagonism in the Mesocortical DA Pathway

FIGURE 2.3. Administration of D2 blockers in the mesocortical pathway, however, is not wanted. Indeed, the hypoactivity of this pathway, which is related to cognitive symptoms (in the DLPFC), negative symptoms (in the DLPFC and VMPFC), and affective symptoms of schizophrenia (in the VMPFC) can actually be worsened by D2 blockade.

As the PFC does not have a high density of D2 receptors, the worsening of negative symptoms might also result from a deficient mesolimbic DA pathway.

In order to treat both positive and negative symptoms it is important to decrease DA activity in the mesolimbic pathway and increase DA tone in the mesocortical pathway. Dopamine function in schizophrenia is not simply "too high" or "too low;" it might be "out of tune." Thus today's psychopharmacologist needs to learn how to tune the system adequately.

D2 Antagonism in the Nigrostriatal DA Pathway

FIGURE 2.4. The nigrostriatal DA pathway, which is an integral part of the extrapyramidal nervous system, regulates motor control. This pathway appears to be relatively spared in schizophrenia; it does, however, induce the motor side effects seen after administration of conventional antipsychotics.

A lack of DA in this pathway results in movement disorders such as rigidity, akinesia, bradykinesia, and tremor, all hallmarks of Parkinson's disease.

A surplus of DA in this pathway, on the other hand, results in hyperkinetic movement disorders such as chorea and dyskinesia. Blockade of D2 receptors, such as with a conventional antipsychotic, prevents DA from binding there and can lead to motor side effects that are often collectively termed extrapyramidal side effects (EPS).

Consequences of Chronic Receptor Blockade

Downregulation

Upregulation

FIGURE 2.5. The rate of synthesis of a receptor is controlled by intracellular enzymes relaying chemical instructions to the cell's DNA. When a protein kinase phosphorylates the transcription factor that tells the cell to slow down the synthesis of the neurotransmitter's receptor, it is called receptor down-regulation. This slowing is exemplified by the red tortoise.

FIGURE 2.6. On the other hand, phosphorylation of a different transcription factor tells the cell to speed up synthesis of the neurotransmitter's receptor. This upregulation, which results in more receptors being expressed on the cell's surface and at a faster pace, is exemplified by the green hare.

Side Effects Due to Chronic D2 Blockade

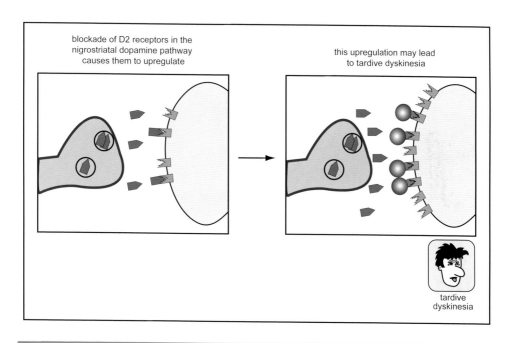

blockade of D2 receptors in the nigrostriatal dopamine pathway causes them to upregulate

this upregulation may lead to tardive dyskinesia

tardive dyskinesia

FIGURE 2.7. Long-term blockade of D2 receptors in the nigrostriatal DA pathway can lead to tardive dyskinesia, a hyperkinetic movement disorder characterized by facial and tongue movements (e.g., tongue protrusions, facial grimaces, chewing) as well as quick, jerky limb movements. Chronic administration of conventional antipsychotics can lead to D2 receptor supersensitivity, or upregulation, where an increase in receptor number attempts to overcome the drug-induced receptor blockade.

Every year, 5% of patients on conventional antipsychotics will develop tardive dyskinesia (25% of patients will be affected by 5 years), and for a disorder that starts in the early 20s, these odds are not acceptable.

Removing the conventional antipsychotic in time can prevent the occurrence of tardive dyskinesia, as this will allow the D2 receptors to lose their sensitivity and downregulate. However, if this is not done in time, irreversible molecular changes take place leading to tardive dyskinesia. Patients developing EPS early in their treatment appear more susceptible to tardive dyskinesia, and need to be monitored closely.

D2 Antagonism in the Tuberoinfundibular DA Pathway

FIGURE 2.8. The tuberoinfundibular DA pathway projects from the hypothalamus to the pituitary gland, and tonically inhibits prolactin release. However, in the postpartum state, decreasing DA activity results in rising prolactin levels facilitating milk production during breast-feeding.

Theoretically, the tuberoinfundibular DA pathway is "normal" in untreated schizophrenia. However, conventional antipsychotics reduce activity in this pathway, allowing prolactin levels to rise. Hyperprolactinemia ensues and is associated with side effects such as galactorrhea (breast secretions) and amenorrhea (irregular menstrual periods), as well as faster demineralization of bones in postmenopausal women. Elevated prolactin levels can also induce sexual dysfunction and weight gain.

Effects of D2 Antagonism on DA Circuitry: Part 1

FIGURE 2.9. In untreated schizophrenia, DA output is high in the mesolimbic pathway, leading to positive symptoms, and low in the mesocortical pathways, leading to negative symptoms (projections to both DLPFC and VMPFC), cognitive symptoms (specifically the projections to the DLPFC), and affective symptoms (especially the projections to the VMPFC).

FIGURE 2.10. A D2 antagonist reduces DA output indiscriminately throughout the brain. While positive symptoms of psychosis will be successfully reduced, the experience of pleasure also mediated by the mesolimbic DA pathway will be impaired. The near shut-down of the mesolimbic DA pathway necessary to improve positive symptoms can lead to anhedonia and apathy. Decreasing DA output in the hypoactive mesocortical pathways will further reduce this pathway's activity and can actually worsen cognitive, negative, or affective symptoms.

Effects of D2 Antagonism on DA Circuitry: Part 2

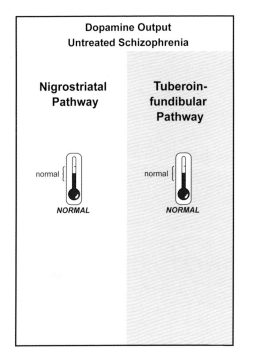

Dopamine Output
Untreated Schizophrenia

Nigrostriatal Pathway

normal { NORMAL

Tuberoin-fundibular Pathway

normal { NORMAL

Dopamine Output - After Pure D2 Antagonist

Nigrostriatal Pathway

normal { LOW

Tuberoin-fundibular Pathway

normal { LOW

parkinsonism

elevated prolactin

FIGURE 2.11. Unlike what is hypothesized for the mesolimbic and mesocortical pathways, DA output is theoretically normal in the nigrostriatal and tuberoinfundibular pathways. Thus, it would make sense that one would not want to alter the normal activity in these pathways when treating schizophrenia.

FIGURE 2.12. By reducing DA output in the nigrostriatal pathway, D2 antagonists can lead to EPS and tardive dyskinesia. Chronic DA blockade of the tuberoinfundibular pathway will result in hyperprolactinemia and its accompanying complications.

Tight and Long-Lasting Binding of Conventional Antipsychotics

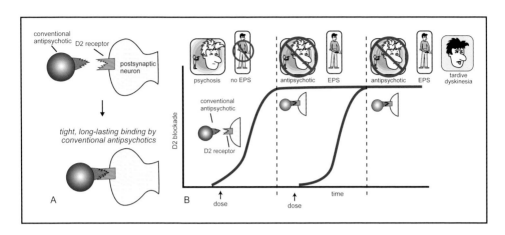

FIGURE 2.13. (A) When conventional antipsychotics bind to D2 receptors, this binding is tight and long-lasting. The teeth on the binding site of the conventional antipsychotic bind tightly to the grooves of the D2 receptor, locking the drug into the receptor binding site and blocking it in a long-lasting manner.

(B) In the absence of D2 receptor blockade, a patient with schizophrenia exhibits positive symptoms of psychosis such as delusions and hallucinations, but does not have EPS. In the presence of a conventional antipsychotic, D2 receptor blockade is very tight, leading to both antipsychotic action and EPS. Following addition of a second dose of a conventional antipsychotic, the D2 receptor blockade remains in place. Thus antipsychotic actions that result from conventional antipsychotics are continuously associated with EPS and can eventually lead to tardive dyskinesia.

Additional Side Effects of Conventional Antipsychotics

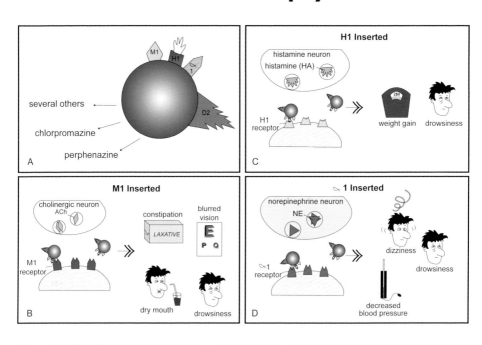

FIGURE 2.14. (A) Besides blockade at D2 receptors, conventional antipsychotics have additional pharmacologic properties: blockade of M1 muscarinic cholinergic receptors, blockade of H1 histamine receptors and blockade of alpha1 adrenergic receptors. These induce side effects common to all drugs with this receptor profile.

(B) The M1 muscarinic anticholinergic portion of the drug can lead to constipation, blurred vision, dry mouth, and drowsiness when binding to acetylcholine receptors.

(C) The H1 histamine portion of the drug can lead to drowsiness and weight gain.

(D) The alpha1 adrenergic portion of the drug can lead to dizziness, decreased blood pressure, and drowsiness.

The Conventional Antipsychotic Haloperidol

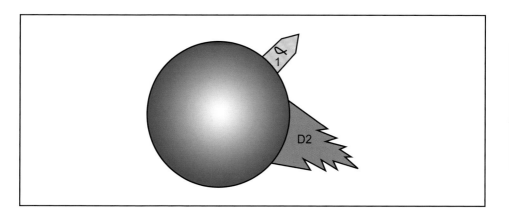

FIGURE 2.15. Haloperidol, one of the most commonly used conventional antipsychotics, has relatively weak cholinergic and histaminergic binding activity but exhibits substantial inhibition at alpha1 adrenergic receptors.

Although they are very efficacious at reducing positive symptoms, conventional antipsychotics are plagued with side effects and thus their use has decreased over time. The propensity of conventional antipsychotics to induce EPS is one of the main reasons that most psychopharmacologists stay away from these medications. However, even within this class of drugs there are differences. Varying degrees of blockade at the muscarinic cholinergic receptors, for example, will lead to different amounts of EPS, such that weak anticholinergic activity induces more EPS and strong anticholinergic activity leads to less severe EPS.

Cholinergic Side Effects of Antipsychotics: Part 1

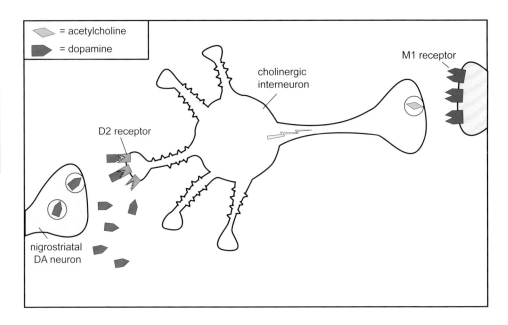

FIGURE 2.16. DA and acetylcholine have a reciprocal relationship in the nigrostriatal DA pathway.

Normally, when DA is released onto cholinergic dendrites it stimulates D2 receptors, and acetylcholine release is suppressed.

Cholinergic Side Effects of Antipsychotics: Part 2

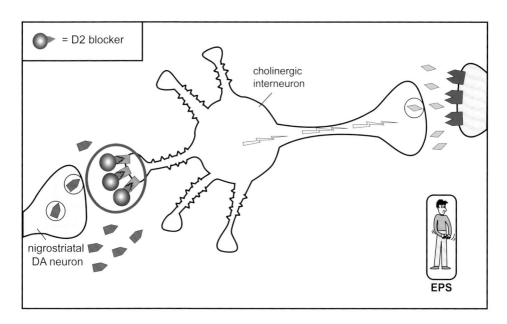

FIGURE 2.17. Blockade of D2 receptors by conventional antipsychotics removes the inhibitory action of DA on the cholinergic neurons (red circle on the left) and leads to increased acetylcholine release (pink acetylcholine on the right). The resulting increased stimulation of postsynaptic cholinergic receptors is correlated with the induction of EPS.

Cholinergic Side Effects of Antipsychotics: Part 3

FIGURE 2.18. Thus it appears that EPS can be induced in a system where DA is low and acetylcholine is high. Blocking the overactive acetylcholine release with an M1 receptor antagonist for example (anticholinergic, circle on the right) will compensate for the increased acetylcholine release induced by D2 receptor blockade. This will thus decrease or prevent the occurrence of EPS.

– SECTION 2 –
Atypical Antipsychotics

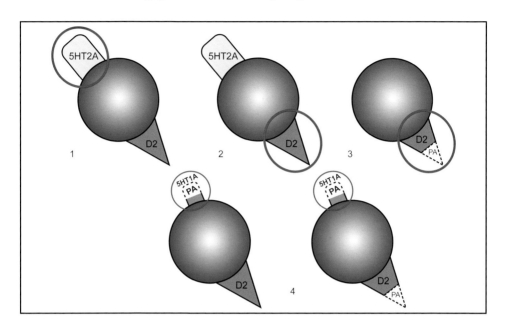

FIGURE 2.19. Atypical antipsychotics represent the second generation of antipsychotics. They are distinguished from conventional antipsychotics by their clinical properties (low EPS and good efficacy for negative symptoms), as well as by four pharmacological characteristics:

(1) Atypical antipsychotics couple their D2 antagonism with 5HT2A antagonism.

(2) The dissociation rate at the D2 receptor sets apart the "atypicality" of an antipsychotic. Tight and long-lasting binding is characteristic of conventional antipsychotics, whereas rapid dissociation is a feature of atypical antipsychotics.

(3) Atypical antipsychotics can also be D2 partial agonists (DPAs). These agents bind in a manner that is neither too antagonizing nor too stimulating, allowing for just the "right" amount of neurotransmission at D2 receptors.

(4) Full or partial agonism at the 5HT1A receptor can also be a characteristic of some atypical antipsychotics. Stimulation at the 5HT1A receptor can increase DA release, thus improving affective, cognitive, and negative symptoms while reducing the risk of EPS and prolactin elevation. Serotonin1A agonism can also decrease glutamate release, which may indirectly reduce the positive symptoms of psychosis.

Rapid Dissociation Theory of Atypical Antipsychotic Action

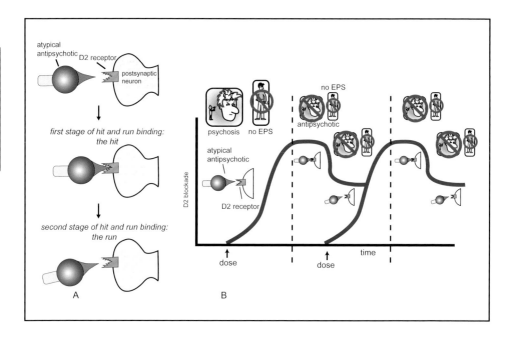

FIGURE 2.20. (A) Unlike conventional antipsychotics, atypical antipsychotics do not have teeth on their binding site, and thus they cannot be locked into position upon binding to D2 receptors. Atypical antipsychotics interact loosely with D2 receptors, exemplified by their smooth binding site. This results in a rapid dissociation from the binding site, also referred to as the "hit and run" receptor binding property. Thus during the "hit," the atypical antipsychotic does not get locked into the receptor binding site and is able to "run" and slip away easily.

(B) An untreated patient with schizophrenia exhibits positive symptoms but no EPS. Upon administration of an atypical antipsychotic, the D2 receptors get blocked for only a short period of time, in contrast to the long-lasting blockade from conventional antipsychotics. Only short blockade of D2 receptors is theoretically required for antipsychotic action, whereas persistent blockade of D2 receptors is required for EPS to occur. Atypical antipsychotics are beneficial in treating the positive symptoms of schizophrenia while preventing EPS, as dose after dose, they bind just long enough to D2 receptors to induce antipsychotic effects, but they "run away" before eliciting EPS.

Effects of Rapid D2 Dissociation on DA Circuitry: Part 1

FIGURE 2.21. In untreated schizophrenia, DA output is high in the mesolimbic pathway, leading to positive symptoms, and low in the mesocortical pathways, leading to negative symptoms (projections to both DLPFC and VMPFC), cognitive symptoms (specifically the projections to the DLPFC), and affective symptoms (especially the projections to the VMPFC).

FIGURE 2.22. Administration of an agent that rapidly dissociates from D2 receptors leads to a reduced DA output in the mesolimbic DA pathway, thus decreasing positive symptoms. Unfortunately, decreasing DA output in this pathway can also lower the experiences of pleasure and reward. Loose binding of atypical antipsychotics in the mesocortical DA pathway could potentially reset this pathway. Theoretically, persistent blockade of D2 receptors is needed in this pathway to worsen affective, cognitive, or negative symptoms. Thus rapid blockade of and dissociation from D2 receptors in the mesocortical pathway may not lead to these side effects.

Effects of Rapid D2 Dissociation on DA Circuitry: Part 2

FIGURE 2.23. Unlike what is hypothesized for the mesolimbic and mesocortical pathways, DA output is theoretically normal in the nigrostriatal and tuberoinfundibular pathways. Thus it would make sense that one would not want to alter the normal activity in these pathways when treating schizophrenia.

FIGURE 2.24. In the nigrostriatal and tuberoinfundibular DA pathways, administration of agents that rapidly dissociate from D2 receptors may exhibit reduced risk for EPS and may not lead to elevated prolactin levels.

Pharmacological Profile of Atypical Antipsychotics

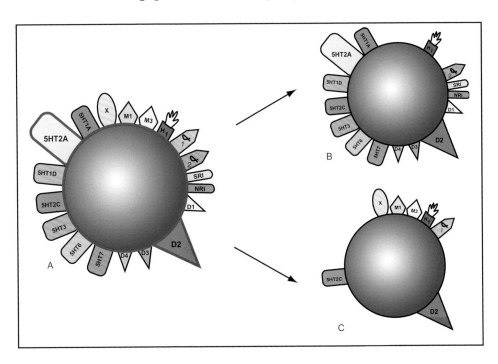

FIGURE 2.25. One characteristic of atypical antipsychotics is their vast pharmacological profile. (A) Besides being D2 and 5HT2A blockers, they interact with more receptors of the DA and 5HT family, such as 5HT1A, 5HT1D, 5HT2C, 5HT3, 5HT6, 5HT7 receptors, the 5HT transporter, and D1, D3 and D4 receptors, and with receptors of other neurotransmitters, such as the norepinephrine transporter and the muscarinic 1 and 3, histamine 1, and alpha 1 and 2 adrenergic receptors. Receptor "X" represents the unclear actions that some atypical antipsychotics have on the insulin system, where they change cellular insulin resistance and increase fasting plasma triglyceride levels.

While some of the different pharmacological properties of atypical antipsychotics contribute to their therapeutic effects (B), others can actually elicit side effects (C).

No two atypical antipsychotics have identical binding properties, which probably helps to explain how they all have somewhat distinctive clinical properties.

Atypical 5HT2A/D2 Antipsychotics: Overview

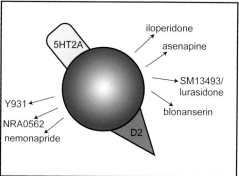

FIGURE 2.26. Presented in this figure are the atypical antipsychotics that are 5HT2A/D2 antagonists, including clozapine, risperidone, paliperidone, olanzapine, quetiapine, and ziprasidone in the United States, as well as perospirone, zotepine, and sertindole in other countries. Loxapine and cyamemazine may also be considered 5HT2A/D2 antagonists when given at low doses.

FIGURE 2.27. New 5HT2A/D2 antagonists are currently in development; these include iloperidone, asenapine, SM13493/lurasidone, blonanserin, nemonapride, NRA0562, and Y931.

Combined 5HT2A/D2 Receptor Blockade Leads to Less EPS

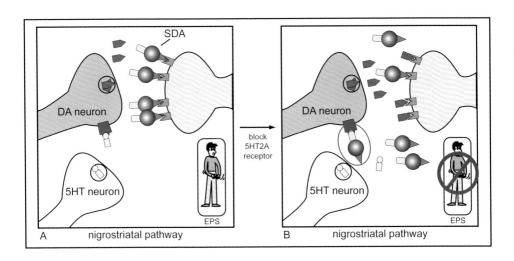

FIGURE 2.28. When postsynaptic D2 receptors are blocked by antagonists, especially long-term, this can result in the occurrence of EPS. This can also occur with 5HT2A/D2 antagonists if only the DA blocking property is active, as represented in (A).

When both D2 and 5HT2A receptors are blocked by SDAs, then the 5HT2A blockade actually opposes the actions of the D2 blockade. Blocking 5HT2A receptors leads to increased DA release, as 5HT normally inhibits DA release (B).

Increased levels of DA in the synapse will then compete with the SDAs for the D2 receptors on the postsynaptic neurons, thus preventing full inhibition. Reversal of D2 blockade therefore prevents the occurrence of EPS, similarly to what is seen in compounds with rapid D2 dissociation.

Effects of 5HT2A Blockade in the Mesocortical DA Pathway

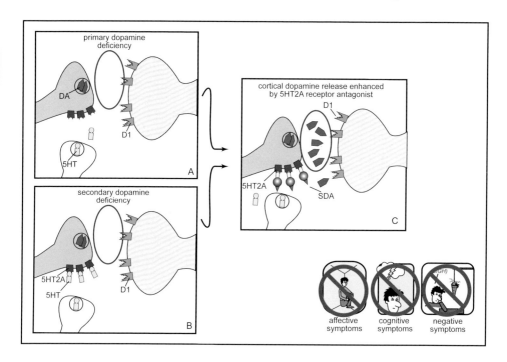

FIGURE 2.29. Affective, cognitive, and negative symptoms are thought to be the result of a lack of DA stimulation in the mesocortical pathway. DA deficiency could be primary (A) or secondary (B) due to excess release of 5HT (5HT inhibits DA release).

Blockade of 5HT2A receptors following administration of SDAs should actually lead to increased synaptic DA levels, which could compensate for the DA deficiency and relieve affective, cognitive, and negative symptoms (C).

Indirect Regulation of Mesolimbic DA Pathway by 5HT2A Blockade in the Cortex

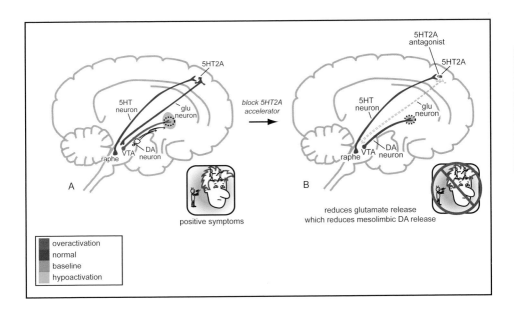

FIGURE 2.30. 5HT2A receptor stimulation can also indirectly regulate DA activity in the mesolimbic DA pathway. 5HT projections from the raphe synapse onto cortical glutamate projections that synapse onto DA projections in the VTA.

(A) Normally, released 5HT stimulates 5HT2A receptors on cortical glutamate projections. This leads to stimulation of these projections and thus excitation of DA neurons in the VTA, possibly resulting in the positive symptoms of schizophrenia.

(B) By blocking 5HT2A receptors in the cortex, glutamate release is reduced in the VTA and thus the excitation of DA neurons in the VTA is also decreased. Antagonizing 5HT2A receptors in the cortex can therefore possibly be used to block the positive symptoms of schizophrenia.

Prolactin Regulation by DA and 5HT

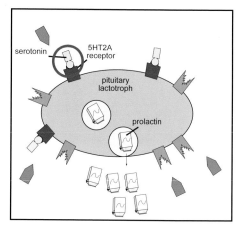

FIGURE 2.31. How do DA and 5HT normally regulate prolactin secretion in the tuberoinfundibular pathway? Under normal conditions, DA is inhibitory to prolactin release from pituitary lactotroph cells by binding to D2 receptors in the pituitary gland (red circle).

FIGURE 2.32. On the other hand, when 5HT binds to 5HT2A receptors on pituitary lactotroph cells, prolactin release is increased (red circle). Thus, 5HT and DA regulate prolactin release in an opposing manner.

Effects of Conventional vs. Atypical 5HT2A/D2 Antipsychotics on Prolactin Release

 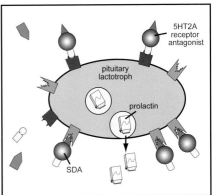

FIGURE 2.33. Due to their antagonism at D2 receptors, conventional antipsychotics block the inhibitory action that DA has on prolactin, and therefore lead to increased prolactin release.

FIGURE 2.34. Atypical antipsychotics such as 5HT2A/D2 antagonists have no net effect on prolactin release and allow normal levels of prolactin to be secreted. Whereas blocking D2 receptors increases prolactin release, blocking 5HT2A receptors blocks the D2-induced release of prolactin. Thus antagonism at one receptor subtype cancels the action of blocking the other receptor, and no net change is observed in prolactin release.

Effects of 5HT2A/D2 Antagonism on DA Circuitry: Part 1

FIGURE 2.35. In untreated schizophrenia, DA output is high in the mesolimbic pathway, leading to positive symptoms, and low in the mesocortical pathways, leading to negative symptoms (projections to both DLPFC and VMPFC), cognitive symptoms (specifically the projections to the DLPFC), and affective symptoms (especially the projections to the VMPFC).

FIGURE 2.36. Administration of a 5HT2A/D2 antagonist decreases the DA output in the mesolimbic DA pathway, thereby reducing the positive symptoms of psychosis. Unfortunately this action may also reduce the experience of pleasure or reward, which is also mediated by that pathway. 5HT2A antagonism can offset a decrease in mesocortical DA resulting from D2 blockade and result in a net increase in DA output in that pathway, thereby treating the cognitive, affective, and negative symptoms of schizophrenia.

Effects of 5HT2A/D2 Antagonism on DA Circuitry: Part 2

FIGURE 2.37. Unlike what is hypothesized for the mesolimbic and mesocortical pathways, DA output is theoretically normal in the nigrostriatal and tuberoinfundibular pathways. Thus it would make sense that one would not want to alter the normal activity in these pathways when treating schizophrenia.

FIGURE 2.38. The net result of blocking 5HT2A and D2 receptors in the nigrostriatal and tuberoinfundibular pathways could be a normalization of the DA output, thus eliminating the risks of the development of EPS and preventing the increase in prolactin levels.

− SECTION 3 −
D2 Partial Agonists

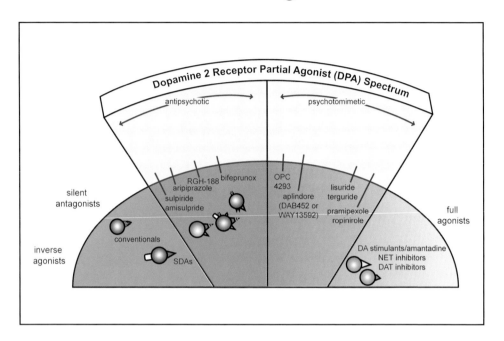

FIGURE 2.39. Atypical antipsychotics also fall within the agonist spectrum, ranging from inverse agonist to full agonist. Some atypical antipsychotics specifically fall within the partial agonist sector of this full agonist spectrum. Too much agonism resembles a psychotomimetic, which is unfavorable in the treatment of schizophrenia.

Partial agonists that lie closer to the antagonist side of the spectrum are favored, and some exhibit good antipsychotic efficacy, such as aripiprazole. Other agents, such as amisulpride and sulpiride, may exhibit partial agonist properties at low doses.

The Agonist Spectrum:
The Theory Behind Partial Agonists

FIGURE 2.40

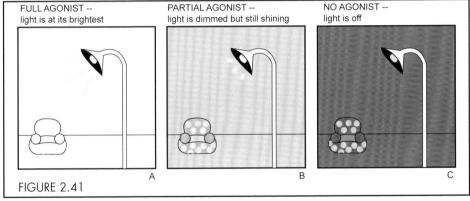

FULL AGONIST --
light is at its brightest

PARTIAL AGONIST --
light is dimmed but still shining

NO AGONIST --
light is off

A

B

C

FIGURE 2.41

FIGURE 2.40. Naturally occurring neurotransmitters that stimulate receptors are agonists; thus drugs that stimulate receptors are also called agonists. Drugs that stimulate a receptor to a lesser degree are partial agonists or stabilizers. Antagonists are "silent" and do not have an action of their own; they only block the action of agonists. Inverse agonists can block the actions of the agonist, or they can reduce baseline activity in the absence of an agonist.

FIGURE 2.41. A light controlled by a rheostat is a good analogy for the concept of the agonist spectrum. The room is brightest when the light is fully on, as after a full agonist (A). A partial agonist will lead to a partially lit room, either by acting as a "net agonist" turning the lights partially on, or by acting as a "net antagonist" and dimming the light of an agonist (B). In the absence of an agonist or partial agonist, the room is dark, and the light is off (C).

The Agonist Spectrum of the Signal Transduction Pathway

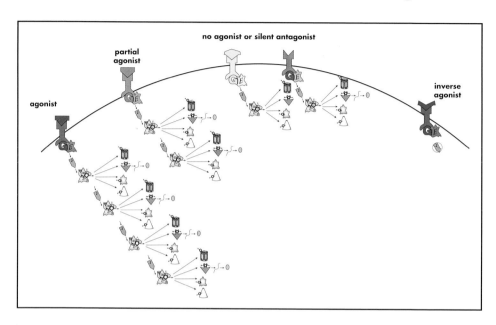

FIGURE 2.42. The concept of the agonist spectrum can also be adapted to the G protein-linked signal transduction system. Whereas a full agonist leads to maximal signal transduction, a partial agonist leads only to a level of signal transduction between the full agonist and no agonist. Antagonists have no effect on signal transduction by themselves, but reduce the level of signal transduction caused by an agonist.

Inverse agonists, on the other hand, can actually lead to lower levels of signal transduction than that which is normally produced in the absence of an agonist.

How Is the DA Spectrum Related to Receptor Output?

FIGURE 2.43. In order to understand the actions of DA and DA agents within an agonist spectrum, it may be helpful to look at them along a "hot-cold" spectrum. That is, DA acts as the ultimate agonist and is too "hot," resulting in psychosis (A). D2 blockers such as conventional antagonists are too "cold," and while they prevent psychotic episodes they also lead to EPS (B). Partial agonists are "lukewarm," leading to just the right stimulation of DA receptors, thus preventing psychotic episodes without inducing EPS (C).

FIGURE 2.44. DA is the ultimate full agonist, leading to full receptor output (A). At the other end of the spectrum, conventional antipsychotics (full antagonists) lead to only very little DA output (B). The atypical antipsychotics that have 5HT2A/D2 blocking activity lead to similarly little DA output. D2 partial agonists (DPAs), on the other hand, stimulate DA receptors only partially, leading to an intermediate or moderate DA output (C).

How Do Partial Agonists Lead to Second Messenger Activation?

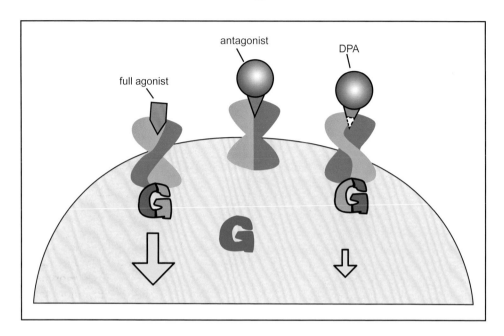

FIGURE 2.45. Similarly the actions of compounds along the agonist spectrum can be seen at the level of the second messenger system. A full agonist results in the full conformational change of the receptor, inducing maximal activation of the G protein-linked signal transduction cascade. An antagonist prevents binding of the G protein to the receptor, and thus prevents second messenger activation. A DA partial agonist results in a conformational change of the receptor leading to partial second messenger activation. The second messenger activation by the partial agonist is only a fraction of the activation resulting from a full agonist.

D2 Partial Agonists: Overview

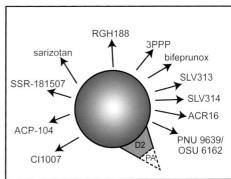

FIGURE 2.46. There is currently one well characterized DA partial agonist (DPA) on the market: aripiprazole. Although not well characterized, amisulpride and sulpiride may also act as partial agonists, especially at low doses.

FIGURE 2.47. DA partial agonists are potentially effective antipsychotics. Many are currently in development, including RGH188, 3PPP, bifeprunox, SLV313, SLV314, ACR16, PNU 9639/ OSU 6162, CI1007, ACP-104, SSR-181507, and sarizotan.

The Benefits of Partial DA Output

FIGURE 2.48. Excessive DA stimulation in the mesolimbic DA pathway theoretically results in psychosis. Similarly to conventional antipsychotics, DA partial agonists block D2 receptors in the mesolimbic DA pathway, thus preventing the excessive DA output from mesolimbic DA neurons that leads to psychosis. Even though DA partial agonists do not reduce DA output as strongly as conventional antipsychotics, their action is sufficient to attain similar antipsychotic efficacy.

FIGURE 2.49. D2 receptor blockade in the nigrostriatal pathway results in EPS. Unlike conventional antipsychotics, DA partial agonists do not completely remove the DA tone in this pathway, thus maintaining normal motor functioning and largely preventing the establishment of EPS.

Effects of D2 Partial Agonism on DA Circuitry: Part 1

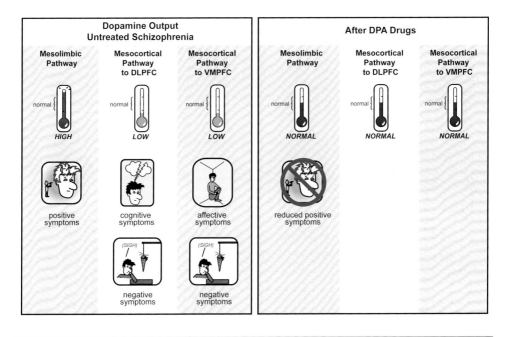

FIGURE 2.50. In untreated schizophrenia, DA output is high in the mesolimbic pathway, leading to positive symptoms, and low in the mesocortical pathways, leading to negative symptoms (projections to both DLPFC and VMPFC), cognitive symptoms (specifically the projections to the DLPFC), and affective symptoms (especially the projections to the VMPFC).

FIGURE 2.51. Administration of a DA partial agonist results in decreased DA output compared to the ultimate agonist, DA. Decreasing DA output in the mesolimbic DA pathway decreases the positive symptoms of psychosis, without affecting the experience of pleasure or reward. In the mesocortical pathways, where DA output is already low in schizophrenia, DA partial agonists may actually increase DA levels, thus improving the cognitive, negative, or affective symptoms of schizophrenia.

Effects of D2 Partial Agonism on DA Circuitry: Part 2

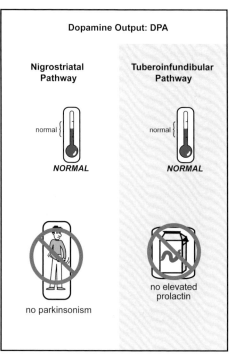

FIGURE 2.52. Unlike what is hypothesized for the mesolimbic and mesocortical pathways, DA output is theoretically normal in the nigrostriatal and tuberoinfundibular pathways. Thus it would make sense that one would not want to alter the normal activity in these pathways when treating schizophrenia.

FIGURE 2.53. In the nigrostriatal and tuberoinfundibular pathways, DA partial agonists should not drastically change DA output. Thus they would not lead to EPS and elevated prolactin levels.

5HT1A Partial Agonism (SPA) of Atypical Antipsychotics

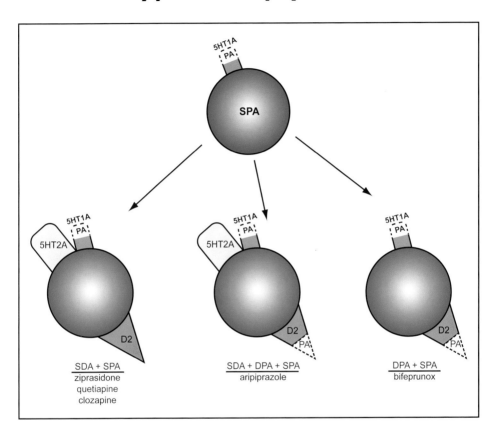

FIGURE 2.54. Various antipsychotics do not fit neatly into a single class of drugs because they combine different receptor actions. Besides being 5HT2A/D2 blockers, ziprasidone, quetiapine, and clozapine are also partial agonists at 5HT1A receptors.

The D2 partial agonist aripiprazole is also an antagonist at 5HT2A receptors and a partial agonist at 5HT1A receptors. Besides being a D2 partial agonist, bifeprunox is also a partial agonist at the 5HT1A receptor.

Chapter 3

Side Effects of Antipsychotics: Metabolic Issues and Sedation

This chapter will go over the metabolic issues and other side effects associated with the different classes of antipsychotics, and explain how an informed psychopharmacologist can ascertain that side effects are minimized and optimal treatment is maximized. Whereas Chapter 4 will expand upon the effects that antipsychotics have on the brain — or the pharmacodynamics of antipsychotics — this chapter includes a section that explains the pharmacokinetics of antipsychotics, namely how brain and body interactions affect the drugs. These are important concepts to understand in order to maximize treatment and minimize side effects.

Which Receptors Can Hypothetically Lead to Cardiometabolic Risk?

FIGURE 3.1. There are a few receptors that, hypothetically, might increase cardiometabolic risk; these include 5HT2C, M3, and H1 receptors, as well as receptors yet to be identified (signified here as receptor "X").

Specifically, 5HT2C and H1 antagonism is linked to weight gain, and M3 receptor antagonism can alter insulin regulation. Receptor "X" may increase insulin resistance, resulting in elevated fasting plasma triglyceride levels. Some patients might be more prone than others to experience increased cardiometabolic risk on certain atypical antipsychotics.

FIGURE 3.2. Simultaneous blockade of 5HT2C and H1 receptors can lead to weight gain, which could result from increased appetite stimulation via hypothalamic eating centers.

Weight Gain and Cardiometabolic Risk of Antipsychotics

Antipsychotic	Weight Gain Risk
Clozapine	+++
Olanzapine	+++
Risperidone*	++
Quetiapine	++
Ziprasidone	+/-
Aripiprazole	+/-

Antipsychotic	Cardiometabolic Risk
Ziprasidone	Low
Aripiprazole	Low
Amisulpride	Possibly low, not well studied
Iloperidone	Possibly low, currently studied
Asenapine	Possibly low, currently studied

* Paliperidone (active metabolite of risperidone) carries the same weight gain risk.
+++ high risk
++ intermediate risk
+/- low risk

TABLE 3.1. Various atypical antipsychotics and their risk of weight gain. The information reflects FDA and expert agreement on three tiers of risk.

TABLE 3.2. Some atypical antipsychotics are "metabolically friendly," in that they are low-risk for both weight gain and cardiometabolic illness.

The Metabolic Highway

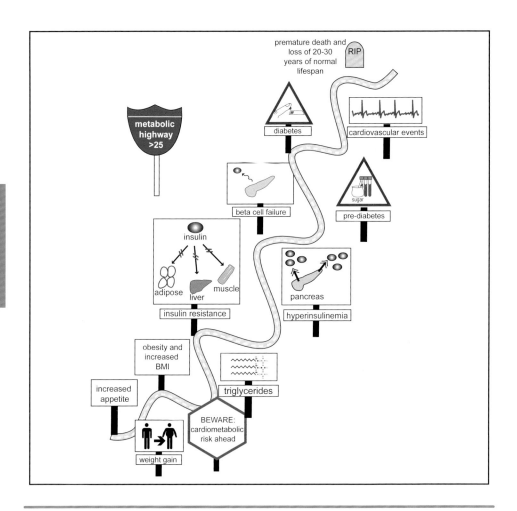

FIGURE 3.3. The metabolic highway depicts different stages that precede cardiovascular disease and premature death. Increased appetite and weight gain combined with a body mass index greater than 25 is the "entrance ramp" to the highway. The highway will eventually lead down the following path: obesity, insulin resistance, and dyslipidemia with increased fasting triglyceride levels.

When hyperinsulinemia leads to pancreatic beta cell failure, pre-diabetes and then diabetes ensue. The presence of diabetes increases a patient's risk for cardiovascular events and premature death.

Insulin Resistance and Antipsychotics

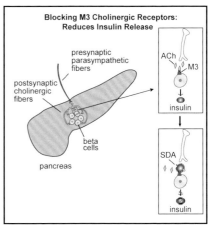

FIGURE 3.4. An unknown pharmacological mechanism is most likely responsible for increased insulin resistance and elevated fasting triglycerides, as seen following the administration of some atypical antipsychotics. In this figure a hypothetical "receptor X" could be the mediator of these actions, allowing atypical antipsychotics to bind to it and leading to insulin resistance of adipose tissue, liver and skeletal muscle.

FIGURE 3.5. Atypical antipsychotics can in rare cases lead to diabetic ketoacidosis (DKA). Normally, insulin secretion is regulated by parasympathetic cholinergic neurons innervating the pancreas and stimulating M3 receptors on pancreatic beta cells. Thus if an atypical antipsychotic has antimuscarinic properties at the M3 receptor, it could potentially lead to reduced insulin release. This could be problematic in patients requiring the cholinergic pathway for the regulation of insulin secretion.

Where on the Metabolic Highway Should Antipsychotic Treatment Be Monitored?

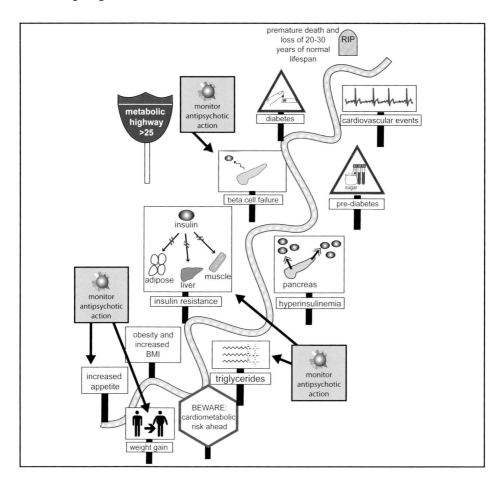

FIGURE 3.6. There are three spots on the metabolic highway that the psychopharmacologist can use to determine whether a patient is "speeding" toward increased cardiometabolic risk when taking different antipsychotics. First, weight gain and body mass index need to be monitored, as both could suggest an increase in appetite and could lead to obesity. Second, fasting triglyceride levels need to be monitored to determine whether the atypical antipsychotic is leading to insulin resistance. Third, it is imperative to educate patients about the symptoms of diabetic ketoacidosis and hyperglycemic hyperosmolar syndrome and to measure fasting glucose levels, as atypical antipsychotics can induce those symptoms suddenly.

Monitoring and Managing Antipsychotics: Best Practices

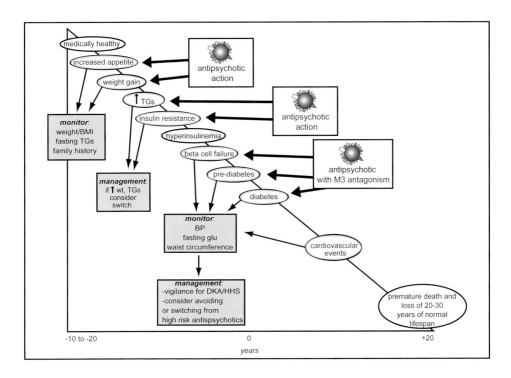

FIGURE 3.7. What are the best practices for monitoring and managing antipsychotics? Patients who will be dosed with atypical antipsychotics should undergo baseline measurements including weight, body mass index (BMI), and fasting triglyceride levels (TGs), and they should provide a family history of diabetes. Weight, BMI, and fasting triglycerides should be monitored throughout treatment, and if weight or triglyceride levels increase, then the patient should be switched to a different antipsychotic, have therapeutic lifestyle interventions, or both.

When patients have dyslipidemia, are pre-diabetic or diabetic, or are obese, it is necessary to obtain their fasting glucose levels, blood pressure and waist circumference measurements just before starting treatment with antipsychotics and throughout treatment. It may be best in these patients to avoid or switch from antipsychotics that exhibit a higher risk of cardiometabolic side effects.

The Involvement of a Psychopharmacologist

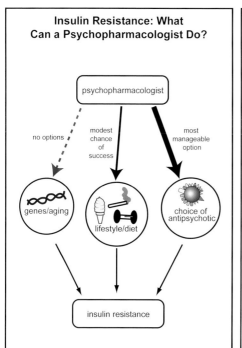

Insulin Resistance: What Can a Psychopharmacologist Do?

psychopharmacologist

no options

modest chance of success

most manageable option

genes/aging

lifestyle/diet

choice of antipsychotic

insulin resistance

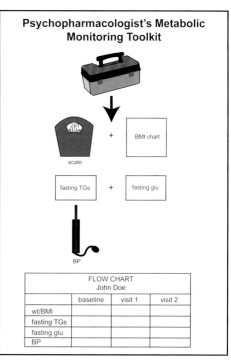

Psychopharmacologist's Metabolic Monitoring Toolkit

scale

+

BMI chart

fasting TGs

+

fasting glu

BP

FLOW CHART John Doe			
	baseline	visit 1	visit 2
wt/BMI			
fasting TGs			
fasting glu			
BP			

FIGURE 3.8. Although a psychopharmacologist can individualize the choice of an atypical antipsychotic, there are various factors that are out of his/her control. These include genetic factors such as age, family history, etc. The psychopharmacologist can also put power into the patients' hands by educating them on lifestyle choices, such as diet, exercise, and smoking. However, the most manageable option for cardiometabolic risk may be which antipsychotic the patient takes.

FIGURE 3.9. A simple metabolic toolkit can be used to track the four main parameters: weight/BMI, fasting triglycerides, fasting glucose and blood pressure. By recording those items at the beginning of treatment and getting regular laboratory tests done for fasting triglycerides and fasting glucose, it is possible to simply monitor a patient and prevent the occurrence of future devastating side effects.

Sedation and Antipsychotics

alpha1 receptors
M1 receptors
H1 receptors

FIGURE 3.10. D2, M1, H1 and alpha1 adrenergic receptor antagonism can all lead to sedation. Thus the atypical antipsychotics with those receptor properties will at some level or another alter arousal in patients.

FIGURE 3.11. Acetylcholine (ACh), histamine (HA), and norepinephrine (NE) are all involved in arousal pathways, thereby connecting neurotransmitter centers with the thalamus (T), hypothalamus (Hy), basal forebrain (BF) and cortex. Thus, it is predictable that atypical antipsychotics with pharmacologic actions that block these receptors could be associated with sedating effects.

Sedation as a Therapeutic Tool

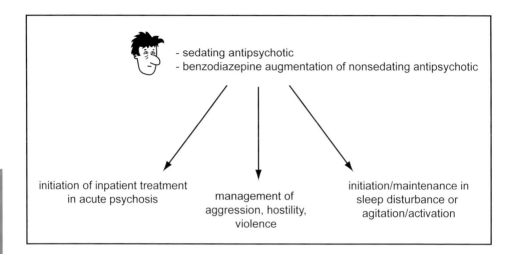

- sedating antipsychotic
- benzodiazepine augmentation of nonsedating antipsychotic

initiation of inpatient treatment in acute psychosis

management of aggression, hostility, violence

initiation/maintenance in sleep disturbance or agitation/activation

FIGURE 3.12. Although it is preferable to avoid long-term sedation, it can be useful initially in the treatment of schizophrenia. Short-term sedation can aid in managing acute psychosis, aggression, hostility, violence, sleep disturbances, or agitation/activation.

A sedating antipsychotic or an adjunct benzodiazepine can be used to induce sedation.

The Reasons for Noncompliance to Antipsychotics

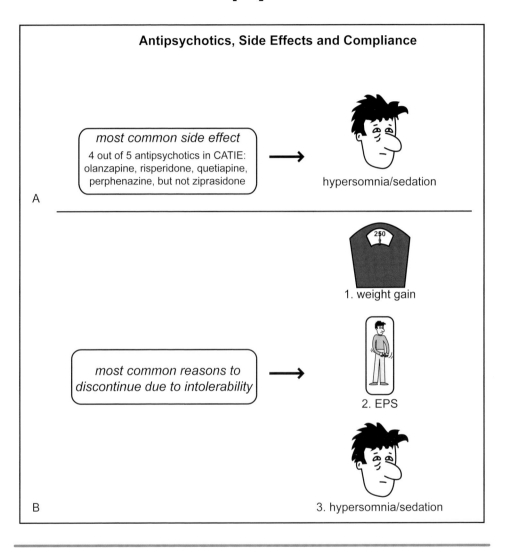

Antipsychotics, Side Effects and Compliance

A

most common side effect
4 out of 5 antipsychotics in CATIE: olanzapine, risperidone, quetiapine, perphenazine, but not ziprasidone

→ hypersomnia/sedation

---

1. weight gain

2. EPS

most common reasons to discontinue due to intolerability

→

B

3. hypersomnia/sedation

FIGURE 3.13. (A) The most common side effect of atypical antipsychotics is sedation, as seen in four of the five antipsychotics studied in the CATIE trial (Clinical Antipsychotic Trials of Intervention Effectiveness). (B) Although short-term sedation can be beneficial, long-term sedation should be avoided. It is among the top three reasons for discontinuing antipsychotic treatment due to intolerability, after weight gain and EPS.

How Can Functional Outcome Be Optimized?

FIGURE 3.14. Blockade of muscarinic M1, histamine H1, and/or alpha1 adrenergic receptors can lead to sedation, which can impact cognitive functioning, attention, memory, and coordination. All of these will result in poor overall functioning for patients with schizophrenia. Somnolence, which can lead to sleepiness and drowsiness, is most likely mediated by blockade of H1 and alpha1 adrenergic receptors. These symptoms can also affect the overall functioning of the patient.

FIGURE 3.15. An adequate treatment of schizophrenia aims to resolve positive symptoms, as well as affective, cognitive, and negative symptoms. Pharmacologically, this requires approximately 70% blockade of D2 receptors in the nucleus accumbens, in addition to antagonism/partial agonism of D2, 5HT2A, and 5HT1A receptors in other key brain regions. Antagonism of histamine H1, muscarinic M1 or alpha 1 adrenergic receptors is best avoided, as these lead to most of the side effects seen with antipsychotics.

The Pathway to Efficacy

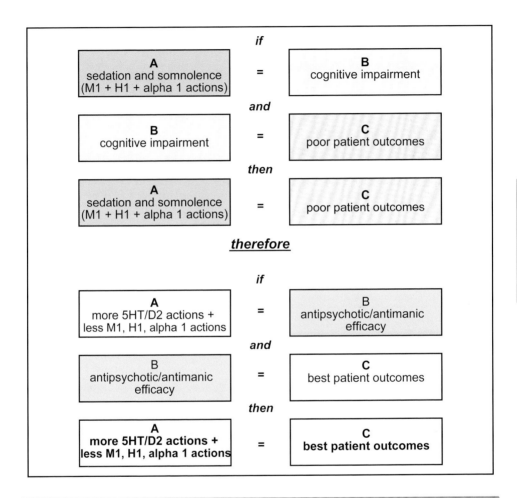

FIGURE 3.16. In order to reach efficacy in the treatment of schizophrenia it is important to ascertain the best possible patient outcome. If blockade of M1, H1 and alpha1 receptors causes sedation and somnolence (which are associated with cognitive impairment), then using antipsychotics with those properties would be related to poor patient outcomes. If, on the other hand, blockade of 5HT and DA receptors has antimanic and antipsychotic efficacy, thus leading to good patient outcome, it would be best to use an antipsychotic that has a 5HT/DA profile, but lacks efficacy at M1, H1, or alpha 1 receptors.

How to Reach the Best Long-Term Outcomes in Schizophrenia?

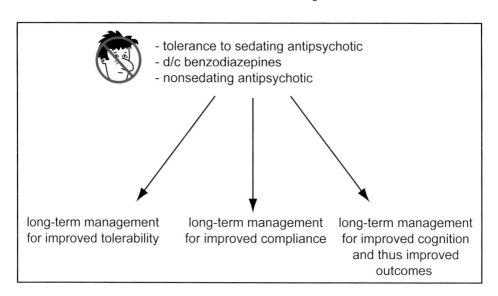

- tolerance to sedating antipsychotic
- d/c benzodiazepines
- nonsedating antipsychotic

long-term management for improved tolerability

long-term management for improved compliance

long-term management for improved cognition and thus improved outcomes

FIGURE 3.17. As one of the top reasons for discontinuing an antipsychotic for intolerability, long-term sedation is best avoided. Patients whose nonsedating antipsychotic medication was initially augmented with a benzodiazepine may need to discontinue the benzodiazepine. For some patients treated with a sedating antipsychotic, it might be necessary to change their medication. Other patients might become tolerant to the sedating side effects of their medication. Careful monitoring to develop individualized treatment is necessary in determining the best possible treatment plan for each patient.

Enzymatic Metabolism of a Drug: The Cytochrome P450 System

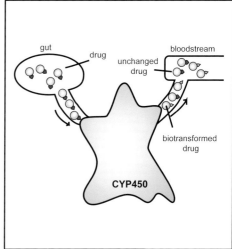

FIGURE 3.18. After a substrate binds to the active site on the enzyme, it is converted into a product which is then released from the enzyme. Some drugs are inhibitors of enzymes; they can either be reversible or irreversible inhibitors. The reversible inhibitor will allow a substrate to compete for the binding site; thus the substrate can reverse the inhibition of the enzyme. In the case of irreversible inhibitors, the substrate cannot displace the inhibitor, and the enzyme essentially becomes unusable. In this case, enzymatic activity is only restored when a new enzyme molecule is synthesized by the cell's DNA.

FIGURE 3.19. The cytochrome P450 (CYP450) enzyme system, which is located in the gut wall and liver, is responsible for the way the body metabolizes drugs such as antipsychotics. When the drug substrate passes through the gut, it is biotransformed into a product released into the bloodstream. Thus upon administration, a drug is partially metabolized by the CYP450 system and partially left unchanged.

Specifics of the CYP450 System

Genetic Polymorphism for Cytochrome P450 2D6

1 in 20

FIGURE 3.20. The cytochrome P450 system encompasses a large number of enzymes. These are classified according to family, subtype, and gene product, using the following nomenclature: 1=family, A=subtype, and 1=gene product. Thus, as depicted in the figure, the five most common and relevant systems are CYP450 1A2, 2D6, 2C9, 2C19, and 3A4.

FIGURE 3.21. Risperidone, clozapine, olanzapine and aripiprazole are all substrates for the cytochrome P450 2D6 enzyme. An individual's genetic make-up determines which CYP450 enzymes s/he has. For example, approximately 1 in 20 Caucasians is a poor metabolizer via 2D6 and thus needs to metabolize drugs by an alternative route. This may (1) not be as metabolically efficient and (2) explain the differential efficacy of various antipsychotics in different patients.

Metabolism of Antipsychotics by CYP450 Enzymes

Drug	Metabolized by
Clozapine	CYP450 1A2, 3A4, 2D6
Risperidone	CYP450 2D6
Paliperidone	Is only weakly metabolized
Olanzapine	CYP450 1A2
Quetiapine	CYP450 3A4, 2D6
Ziprasidone	Not affected by CYP450 enzymes
Aripiprazole	CYP450 3A4, 2D6
Zotepine	CYP450 1A2, 3A4
Perospirone	CYP450 3A4
Sertindole	CYP450 3A4, 2D6
Loxapine	Unknown
Cyamemazine	Unknown
Amisulpride	Is only weakly metabolized
Sulpiride	Is only weakly metabolized
Bifeprunox	CYP450 2C9, 3A4, only little 2D6
Iloperidone	CYP450 3A4, 2D6
Asenapine	CYP450 1A2, 3A4

TABLE 3.3. The hepatic enzymes involved in the metabolism of the 17 antipsychotics described in Chapter 4.

Importance of the CYP450 1A2 Enzyme

FIGURE 3.22. As different drug classes are substrates for different CYP450 enzymes, it is important to understand drug interactions. The antipsychotics clozapine, olanzapine, and zotepine are substrates for cytochrome P450 1A2. If these are given in combination with an antidepressant such as fluvoxamine, which acts as an inhibitor of this enzyme, plasma levels can rise. Thus it is important to know which drugs a patient is taking and to be prepared for the need to adjust dosages.

FIGURE 3.23. Patients with schizophrenia are known to self-medicate by smoking cigarettes. Smoking can induce the enzyme cytochrome P450 1A2, so that the plasma levels of drugs metabolized by this enzyme such as olanzapine, clozapine, and zotepine are lowered. Smokers may therefore need higher levels of these three drugs compared to non-smokers.

Importance of the CYP450 2D6 Enzyme

FIGURE 3.24. Risperidone, clozapine, olanzapine and aripiprazole are substrates for the cytochrome P450 2D6 enzyme. This enzyme often hydroxylates its substrates.

Various antidepressants such as paroxetine, fluoxetine, duloxetine and high doses of sertraline are inhibitors of cytochrome P450 2D6; thus they could theoretically raise the levels of the previously mentioned antipsychotics as these are substrates for the same enzyme. However, this is not usually clinically significant.

FIGURE 3.25. Risperidone is metabolized to paliperidone by the enzyme cytochrome P450 2D6. This active metabolite has been approved as a new antipsychotic.

Importance of the CYP450 3A4 Enzyme

FIGURE 3.26. (A) Clozapine, quetiapine, ziprasidone, sertindole, aripiprazole, and zotepine are substrates for cytochrome P450 3A4. (B) Powerful inhibitors of cytochrome P450 3A4 include the antifungal ketoconazole, some protease inhibitors, the antibiotic erythromycin, and the following antidepressants: fluvoxamine, nefazodone, fluoxetine and its metabolite norfluoxetine.

In the presence of these inhibitors, plasma levels of antipsychotics will be elevated, and thus might need to be adjusted.

FIGURE 3.27. (A) Besides being a substrate or an inhibitor of a cytochrome P450 enzyme, drugs can also be inducers of the system. The mood stabilizer carbamazepine is one such example. The presence of carbamazepine increases the metabolism of the substrates of the 3A4 enzyme, thus requiring higher doses of the substrates. (B) At the same time, if a patient who was taking, for example, carbamazepine in combination with clozapine (a substrate for 3A4) was discontinuing the mood stabilizer, it would be necessary to adjust the dose of the antipsychotic as well. As the autoinduction of 3A4 by carbamazepine would be reversed over time, the original dose of an antipsychotic would be too high.

Seventeen Antipsychotic Drugs

This chapter will describe each antipsychotic medication currently available in terms of side effect profile, dosing tips and drug interactions. As with all atypical antipsychotics discussed in this chapter, binding properties vary greatly with technique and from one laboratory to another; they are constantly being revised and updated. Thus it is important to remain up-to-date on the specifics of each antipsychotic.

Symbols Used in this Chapter			
	Life-threatening or dangerous side effects		Drug Interactions
	Tips and Pearls		Cardiac Impairment
	Children and Adolescents		Renal Impairment
	Pregnancy		Hepatic Impairment

Clozapine

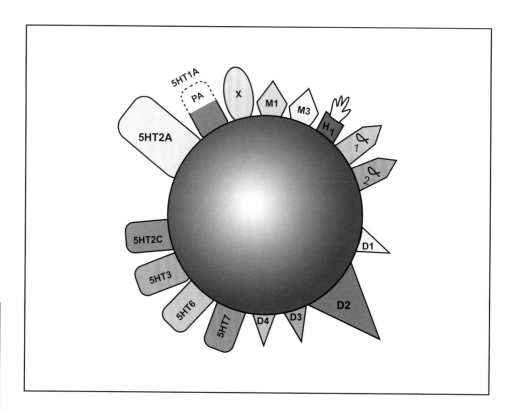

FIGURE 4.1. The most complex receptor profile belongs to clozapine. It has been considered the "prototypical" atypical antipsychotic and leads to few EPS, does not result in tardive dyskinesia and does not elevate prolactin levels. It has proven particularly efficacious when other antipsychotics fail.

Even though it is very effective, clozapine is not considered a first-line agent as it can lead to the potentially life-threatening side effect agranulocytosis. Weight increase and the concomitant risk of developing metabolic complications are greatest with clozapine.

Clozapine: Tips and Pearls

Dosing
Formulation: 12.5, 25, 50 and 100 mg tablets; 12.5, 25, 50 and 100 mg orally disintegrating tablets **Dosage Range:** 300-450 mg/day **Approved For:** Treatment-resistant schizophrenia; reduction in risk of recurrent suicidal behavior in patients with schizophrenia or schizoaffective disorder

Pearls	
	Rapid discontinuation can lead to rebound psychosis; most efficacious but most dangerous; reduces suicide in schizophrenia
	Potentially efficacious in early-onset treatment-resistant schizophrenia; children and adolescents should be monitored more often than adults
	Pregnancy risk category B (animal studies do not show adverse effects, no controlled studies in humans)

Side effects I

Weight Gain

unusual   not unusual   common   problematic

Sedation

unusual   not unusual   common   problematic

	Hyperglycemia, ketoacidosis, agranulocytosis, rare neuroleptic malignant syndrome, increased risk of death in elderly, seizures, myocarditis

Side effects II	
	CYP450 1A2, 3A4 and 2D6 inhibitors increase its plasma levels; CYP450 1A2 inducers decrease its levels; drug enhances effects of antihypertensives
	Use with caution, especially if patient takes concomitant medications
	Use with caution in patients with renal impairments
	Use with caution in patients with hepatic impairments

FIGURE 4.2. Dosing and interaction information for clozapine.

Risperidone

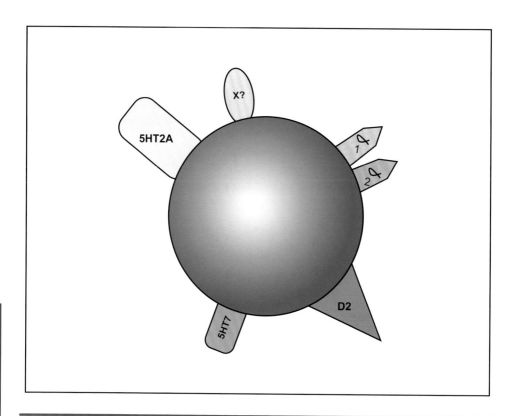

FIGURE 4.3. The receptor profile for risperidone is certainly simpler than the one for clozapine. Risperidone is mostly a 5HT2A/D2 antagonist. At low doses risperidone behaves like an atypical antipsychotic, but if the doses are pushed it can, similarly to conventional drugs, lead to EPS. Risperidone is approved for use in children and adolescents for the following disorders: irritability associated with autistic disorder (ages 5 to 16), bipolar disorder (ages 10 to 17) and schizophrenia (ages 13 to 17).

Risperidone is also available as an intramuscular, long-term depot formulation that lasts two weeks. Risperidone does increase prolactin levels, but there appears to be less risk of weight gain with risperidone, as well as less cardiometabolic risk than with some other atypical antipsychotics, at least in some patients.

Risperidone: Tips and Pearls

Dosing

Formulation:
0.25, 0.5, 1, 2, 3, 4 and 6 mg tablets; 0.5, 1 and 2 mg orally disintegrating tablets; 1mg/mL liquid; 25, 37.5 and 50 mg vial/kit IM depot

Dosage Range:
2-8 mg/day oral (psychosis); 0.5-2 mg/day oral (children and elderly); 25-50 mg depot every 2 weeks

Approved For:
Schizophrenia, delaying relapse in schizophrenia, other psychotic disorders, acute mania/mixed mania

Pearls

 Less may be more; good treatment for agitation (elderly) and behavioral symptoms (children); dose-dependent EPS; less weight gain and sedation than other drugs

 Approved for autism-related irritability (ages 5 to 16), bipolar (ages 10 to 17), schizophrenia (ages 13 to 17)

 Pregnancy risk category C (some animal studies show adverse effects; no controlled studies in humans)

Side effects I

Weight Gain

unusual — not unusual — common — problematic

Sedation

unusual — not unusual — common — problematic

 Hyperglycemia, ketoacidosis and coma, rare neuroleptic malignant syndrome, rare seizures, increased risk of death in elderly

Side effects II

 CYP450 2D6 inhibitors can increase its plasma levels; drug increases effects of antihypertensives and decreases DA agonist effects

 Use with caution in elderly with atrial fibrillation

 In patients with renal impairments, only use long-acting depot if patient tolerates oral formulation

 In patients with hepatic impairments, only use long-acting depot if patient tolerates oral formulation

FIGURE 4.4. Dosing and interaction information for risperidone.

Paliperidone

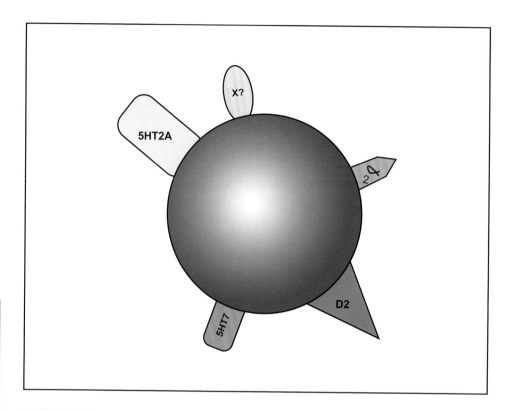

FIGURE 4.5. Paliperidone, also a 5HT2A/D2 antagonist, is the active metabolite of risperidone, and thus has a similar receptor profile. The oral sustained-release formulation of paliperidone allows it to be taken just once a day. This property will most likely also lead to less EPS and sedation compared to its parent compound.

Paliperidone may improve depression due to its alpha 2 antagonist properties. It might however be associated with weight gain, insulin resistance, and diabetes as well as prolactin elevation, similarly to risperidone.

Paliperidone: Tips and Pearls

	Dosing

Formulation:
3, 6, 9 and 12 mg tablets; prolonged-release formulation

Dosage Range:
3-15 mg/day; 6 mg/day has shown optimum efficacy; no titration required

Approved For:
Acute and maintenance treatment of schizophrenia

Pearls	
	Dose-dependent risk of EPS; may elevate prolactin levels and cause weight gain (especially at higher doses); beneficial for people with liver disease or for people on antidepressant (as no interaction with CYP450 enzyme)
	Preliminary study suggests efficacy in children and adolescents
	As with any new drug, it is best to stop when pregnant or when breast-feeding

Side effects I

Weight Gain

Sedation

	Rare neuroleptic malignant syndrome, QTc prolongation, syncope, hyperprolactinemia and akathisia

Side effects II

	Not metabolized by the liver, therefore low potential for interactions with other drugs; advantageous in people with hepatic insufficiency
	Use with caution in patients with cardiac impairments
	Use with caution in patients with renal impairments
	Not metabolized by liver

FIGURE 4.6. Dosing and interaction information for paliperidone.

Olanzapine

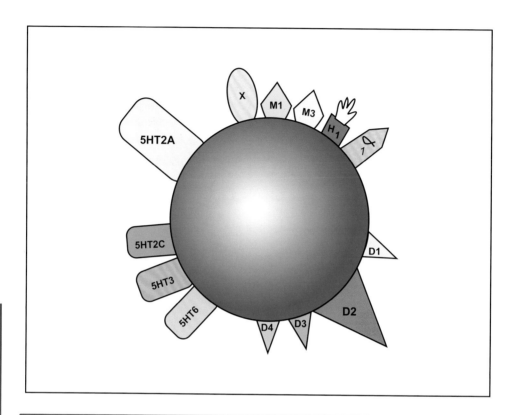

FIGURE 4.7. Olanzapine is a 5HT2A/ D2 antagonist whose chemical structure is very similar to that of clozapine. Even at high doses, olanzapine only induces mild EPS, emphasizing its atypical nature. Even though olanzapine has M1, H1 and alpha 1 antagonistic properties it is not as sedating as clozapine. It is one of the antipsychotics with the greatest cardiometabolic risk, as it leads to weight gain, increased fasting triglyceride levels, and increased insulin resistance.

Olanzapine is often used at doses higher than what the packet insert suggests, as it often exhibits better efficacy and effectiveness at higher doses. Olanzapine appears to be effective at reducing affective and cognitive symptoms, a property most likely related in part to its 5HT2C antagonism. Olanzapine comes in different formulations, including oral disintegrating tablets and intramuscular formulations.

Olanzapine: Tips and Pearls

 Dosing

Formulation:
2.5, 5, 7.5, 10, 15 and 20 mg tablets; 5, 10, 15 and 20 mg orally disintegrating tablets; 5 mg/mL IM formulation; olanzapine/fluoxetine (O/F) combo capsules (6 mg/25 mg; 6 mg/50 mg, 12 mg/25 mg, 12 mg/50 mg)

Dosage Range:
10-20 mg/day (oral or IM); O/F combo: 6-12 mg olanzapine/ 25-50 mg fluoxetine

Approved For:
Schizophrenia (maintenance of it and bipolar), acute agitation (IM), acute and mixed mania, bipolar depression (O/F combo)

Side effects I

Weight Gain

unusual — not unusual — common — problematic

Sedation

unusual — not unusual — common — problematic

 Hyperglycemia, diabetic ketoacidosis, rare seizures, rare neuroleptic malignant syndrome, increased risk of death in elderly, may increase risk for diabetes and dyslipidemia

Pearls

 More may be more; doses above 15 mg/day useful for acutely ill/agitated patients; IM formulation can be given to initiate oral dosing; rapid onset without titration

 Not recommended for use under age 18, but often used, as appears safe and efficacious

 Pregnancy risk category C (some animal studies show adverse effects; no controlled studies in humans)

Side effects II

 CYP450 1A2 inhibitors increase and CYP450 1A2 inducers decrease its plasma levels; drug increases effects of antihypertensives and decreases DA agonist effects

 Use with caution in patients with cardiac impairments

 May need to lower dose in patients with renal impairments

 No dose adjustment needed for oral dose in patients with hepatic impairments; start lower for IM formulation

FIGURE 4.8. Dosing and interaction information for olanzapine.

Quetiapine

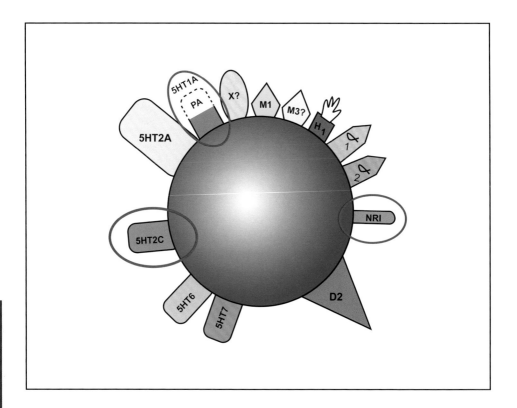

FIGURE 4.9. The 5HT2A/D2 antagonist quetiapine is chemically related to clozapine. Its active metabolite, norquetiapine, has unique features (red circles) that most likely add to quetiapine's efficacy. This very atypical antipsychotic exhibits rapid D2 dissociation, and therefore hardly any EPS and no prolactin elevation. The partial 5HT1A agonist feature of quetiapine and the norepinephrine reuptake-inhibiting and 5HT2C-blocking properties of norquetiapine are most likely responsible for its effectiveness at treating mood and cognitive disorders.

Quetiapine is effective as a once-daily dose, and if given in the evening it will not induce daytime sedation. At moderate to high doses, both quetiapine and norquetiapine can induce weight gain due to histamine H1 blockade and 5HT2C blockade, respectively. Additionally, at these doses, quetiapine can increase triglyceride levels and insulin resistance, emphasizing the need to monitor patients if they are started on this atypical antipsychotic.

Quetiapine: Tips and Pearls

Dosing	Pearls

Formulation:
25, 50, 100, 200, 300 and 400 mg tablets
XR formulation: 200, 300 and 400 mg/day once daily

Dosage Range:
150-750 mg/day (in 2 doses) for schizophrenia, 400-800 mg/day (in 2 doses) for acute bipolar mania 300-600 mg (in 1 dose at bedtime) for bipolar depression

Approved For:
Schizophrenia and maintenance of schizophrenia, acute mania, depressive episodes of bipolar disorder

Pearls

 More may be much more: is often underdosed, but even low doses can be sedating; no motor side effects; no prolactin elevation

 Not recommended for use under age 18, but often used, as appears safe and efficacious; may require lower doses than adults

 Pregnancy risk category C (some animal studies show adverse effects; no controlled studies in humans)

Side effects I

Weight Gain

unusual   not unusual   common   problematic

Sedation

unusual   not unusual   common   problematic

 Hyperglycemia, diabetic ketoacidosis, rare neuroleptic malignant syndrome, seizures, may increase risk for diabetes and dyslipidemia

Side effects II

 CYP450 3A4 and 2D6 inhibitors raise its levels, but dosage adjustment not necessary; drug increases effects of antihypertensives

 Use with caution; orthostatic hypotension possible

 Downward dose adjustment may be needed in patients with renal impairments

 No dose adjustment needed in patients with hepatic impairments

---

FIGURE 4.10. Dosing and interaction information for quetiapine.

Ziprasidone

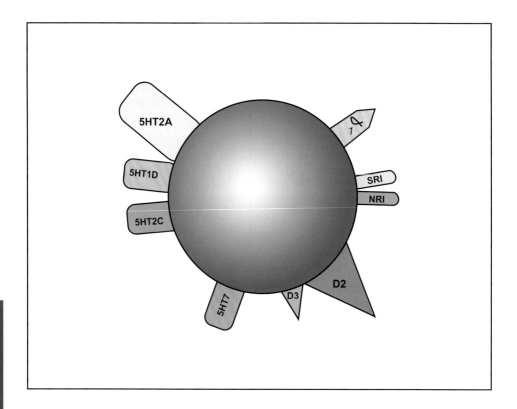

FIGURE 4.11. Compared to the atypical antipsychotics presented so far, ziprasidone is a chemically different compound with interesting pharmacology. Due to its 5HT2A/D2 blocking capability, it reduces the risk of EPS and elevated prolactin levels. Ziprasidone has been shown to treat both positive and negative symptoms. In cases of acute psychosis, the intramuscular formulation is highly effective. Rapid dose escalation to middle to high doses has been proven most effective. Ziprasidone's most differentiating feature is that is does not induce weight gain, dyslipidemia, elevation of fasting triglycerides, or insulin resistance.

The 5HT1D antagonist actions combined with the 5HT and NE reuptake blocking properties might contribute to the absence of weight gain induction by ziprasidone, as well as its potential antidepressant and anxiolytic properties.

Ziprasidone: Tips and Pearls

	Dosing

Formulation:
20, 40, 60 and 80 mg capsules;
20 mg/mL injection

Dosage Range:
40-200 mg/day orally in divided
doses (must be given with food),
10-20 mg intramuscularly

Approved For:
Schizophrenia, delaying relapse in
schizophrenia, acute agitation in
schizophrenia (IM), acute mania/
mixed mania

Pearls

	It is often underdosed; activation occurs at 20-40 mg 2X/day and is reduced at 60-80 mg 2X/day; food doubles bioavailability
	Not recommended for use under age 18, but clinically proven safe and effective
	Pregnancy risk category C (some animal studies show adverse effects; no controlled studies in humans)

Side effects I

Weight Gain

unusual   not unusual   common   problematic

Sedation

unusual   not unusual   common   problematic

	Rare neuroleptic malignant syndrome, rare seizures, increased risk of death in elderly, QTc prolongation

Side effects II

	Not affected by CYP450 enzymes; drug increases effects of antihypertensives and decreases DA agonist effects; may enhance QTc prolongation of other drugs that enhance QTc prolongation
	Contraindicated in patients with QTc prolongation
	No dose adjustment necessary in patients with renal impairments
	No dose adjustment necessary in patients with hepatic impairments

FIGURE 4.12. Dosing and interaction information for ziprasidone.

Aripiprazole

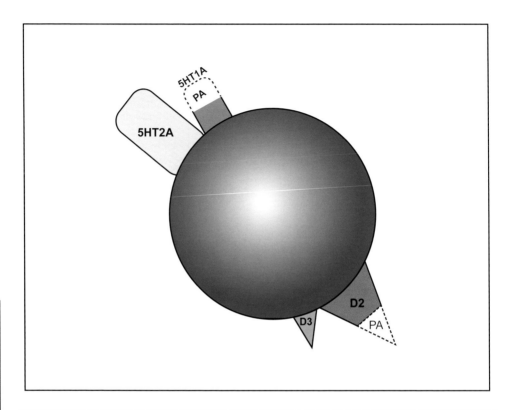

FIGURE 4.13. Aripiprazole is the first atypical antipsychotic with D2 partial agonist properties. Its 5HT2A and 5HT1A features may be the reason for its increased tolerability and efficacy. Aripiprazole is effective at treating positive and manic symptoms. Its benefits also lie in its many different formulations (tablets, disintegrating tablets, liquid and IM formulations). Aripiprazole is usually devoid of sedative side effects, and can even be activating. For some patients aripiprazole is either too close to a full antagonist, or too close to a full agonist. In both cases, dose adjustment and the timing of administration can ameliorate these symptoms.

Similarly to ziprasidone, aripiprazole causes little to no weight gain, most likely because it lacks 5HT2C and histamine H1 properties. Additionally, aripiprazole does not seem to induce dyslipidemia, increase fasting triglyceride levels, or increase insulin resistance. Thus aripiprazole has a lower cardiometabolic risk.

Aripiprazole: Tips and Pearls

 Dosing

Formulation:
2, 5, 10, 15, 20, 30 mg tablets;
1mg/mL oral solution; 10 and 15
mg orally disintegrating tablets;
9.75 mg/1.3 mL single-dose vial
injection

Dosage Range:
15-30 mg/day; solution doses can
be substituted for tablet doses on a
mg-per-mg basis up to 25 mg

Approved For:
Schizophrenia (adults and adolescents), maintaining stability
in schizophrenia, acute mania/
mixed mania, bipolar maintenance;
adjunctive treatment to antidepressants for Major Depressive Disorder
in adults

Pearls

 May be activating; no
diabetes or dyslipidemia risk;
favorable tolerability profile;
for some, less may be more,
for others more may be more

 Not recommended for use
under age 13; approved for
schizophrenia (age 13 to 17)
and bipolar (age 10 to 17)

 Pregnancy risk category C
(some animal studies show
adverse effects; no controlled
studies in humans)

Side effects I

Weight Gain

unusual	not unusual	common	problematic

Sedation

unusual	not unusual	common	problematic

Rare neuroleptic ma-
lignant syndrome, rare
seizures, increased risk
of death in elderly

Side effects II

 CYP450 3A4 or 2D6 inhibitors increase its plasma levels,
and CYP450 3A4 inducers
lower them; drug increases effects of antihypertensives and
decreases DA agonist effects

 Use with caution due to risk of
orthostatic hypotension

 No dose adjustment needed
in patients with renal impairments

 No dose adjustment needed in
patients with hepatic impairments

FIGURE 4.14. Dosing and interaction
information for aripiprazole.

Zotepine

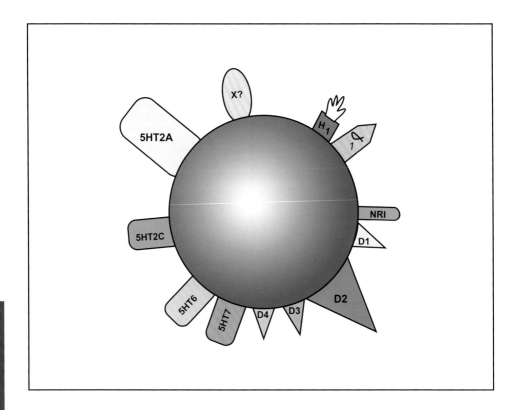

FIGURE 4.15. This 5HT2A/D2 antagonist has a chemical structure similar to that of clozapine, but different pharmacology. Despite its 5HT2A antagonism it can lead to EPS and elevation of prolactin levels. It might also induce weight gain and sedation, and it probably increases the risk for insulin resistance, dyslipidemia, and diabetes.

Another side effect of zotepine is its tendency to increase QTc prolongation. Due to its norepinephrine reuptake inhibition, zotepine has the potential for antidepressant actions.

Zotepine: Tips and Pearls

	Dosing

Formulation:
25, 50 and 100 mg tablets

Dosage Range:
75-300 mg/day in 3 divided doses

Approved For:
Not available in the USA

Pearls	
	Inhibits NE uptake, thus possibly efficacious for cognitive and mood symptoms
	Not recommended for use under age 18
	Not recommended during pregnancy or breast-feeding; insufficient data in humans

Side effects I

Weight Gain

unusual   not unusual   common   problematic

Sedation

unusual   not unusual   common   problematic

	Blood dyscrasias, rare neuroleptic malignant syndrome, rare seizures, increases risk of death in elderly, dose-dependent QTc prolongation, hyperglycemia, diabetic ketoacidosis, increases risk for diabetes and dyslipidemia

Side effects II

	CYP450 1A2 and 3A4 inhibitors increase its plasma levels, CYP450 1A2 inducers (cigarette smoking) lower them
	Use with caution as it dose-dependently increases QTc prolongation
	Best to start at 25 mg 2X/day, max dose of 75 mg 2X/day in patients with renal impairments
	Best to start at 25 mg 2X/day, max dose of 75 mg 2X/day in patients with hepatic impairments

FIGURE 4.16. Dosing and interaction information for zotepine.

Perospirone

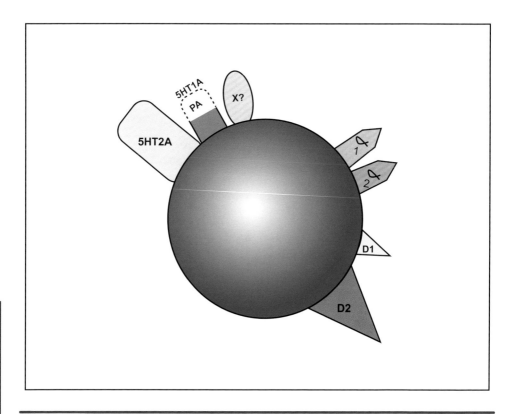

FIGURE 4.17. Perospirone is a 5HT2A/ D2 antagonist with 5HT1A partial agonist properties, which most likely contribute to its efficacy. Its side effect profile has not been well established.

Perospirone: Tips and Pearls

 Dosing

Formulation:
4 and 8 mg tablets

Dosage Range:
8-48 mg/day in 3 divided doses

Approved For:
Schizophrenia (in Japan); not available in the USA

Pearls

 Interactions at 5HT1A receptors suggest possible efficacy for depression and anxiety symptoms, might have worse EPS than other atypical antipsychotics

 Use with caution in children and adolescents

 Recommended to discontinue drug during pregnancy or breast-feeding

Side effects I

Weight Gain
> **Not well characterized**

Sedation

unusual   not unusual   common   problematic

 Rare neuroleptic malignant syndrome, increased risk of death in elderly

Side effects II

 CYP450 3A4 inhibitors increase its plasma levels; CYP450 3A4 inducers decrease its plasma levels

 Use with caution in patients with cardiac impairments

 Use with caution in patients with renal impairments

 Use with caution in patients with hepatic impairments

FIGURE 4.18. Dosing and interaction information for perospirone.

Sertindole

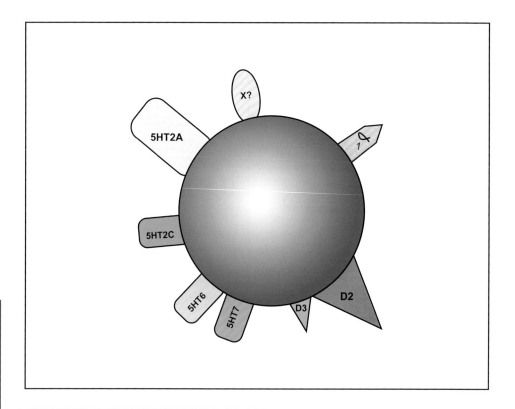

FIGURE 4.19. Another atypical antipsychotic with a 5HT2A/D2 antagonism profile is sertindole. It has proven beneficial in patients not responding to other treatment; however, patients need to be closely monitored for their cardiac status and drug interactions, as sertindole can increase QTc prolongation.

Sertindole: Tips and Pearls

Dosing
Formulation: 4, 12, 16 and 20 mg tablets
Dosage Range: 12-20 mg/day, can go up to 24 mg/day
Approved For: Not available in the USA

Pearls	
	Has been shown to reduce negative symptoms
	Efficacy and safety unknown in children and adolescents
	Recommended to stop treatment during pregnancy or breast-feeding

Side effects I	
Weight Gain unusual / not unusual / common / problematic	
Sedation unusual / not unusual / common / problematic	
	QTc prolongation

Side effects II	
	CYP450 2D6 and 3A4 inhibitors increase its plasma levels, and inducers decrease its plasma levels
	Use with caution due to possible QTc prolongation
	Use with caution in patients with renal impairments
	Use caution in patients with hepatic impairments

FIGURE 4.20. Dosing and interaction information for sertindole.

Loxapine:
Conventional or Low-Dose Atypical?

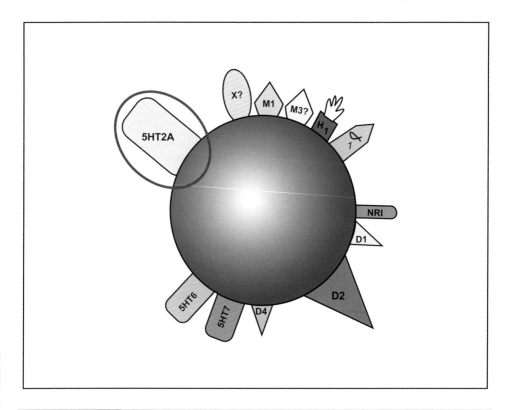

FIGURE 4.21. Although loxapine has a chemical structure similar to that of clozapine and exhibits 5HT2A/D2 antagonism, it is often classified as a conventional antipsychotic, as it can lead to EPS and prolactin elevation. Apparently, however, low doses of loxapine can be more "atypical."

Although loxapine usually does not lead to weight gain, it might present a cardiometabolic risk. Loxapine has an intramuscular formulation, and its metabolite amoxapine is a tricyclic antidepressant.

Loxapine: Tips and Pearls

Dosing

Formulation:
6.8 mg, 13.6 mg, 34 mg and 68.1 mg loxapine succinate capsules (equivalent of 5, 10, 25, 50 mg loxapine, respectively); 25 mg/mL oral liquid; 50 mg/mL injection

Dosage Range:
60-100 mg/day in divided doses

Approved For:
Schizophrenia

Pearls

May be an atypical antipsychotic at lower doses; one active metabolite is an antidepressant (amoxapine)

Safety and efficacy not established in children and adolescents, 2nd-line treatment after atypical antipsychotic

Not recommended during pregnancy or breast-feeding; insufficient data in humans

Side effects I

Weight Gain

unusual | not unusual | common | problematic

Sedation

unusual | not unusual | **common** | problematic

Rare neuroleptic malignant syndrome, rare seizures, increased risk of death in elderly, rare hepatocellular injury, rare agranulocytosis, galactorrhea

Side effects II

In combo with lorazepam induces respiratory depression; decreases effects of DA agonists; decreases BP in combo with epinephrine

Use with caution in patients with cardiac impairments

Use with caution in patients with renal impairments

Use with caution in patients with hepatic impairments

FIGURE 4.22. Dosing and interaction information for loxapine.

Cyamemazine:
Conventional or Low-Dose Atypical?

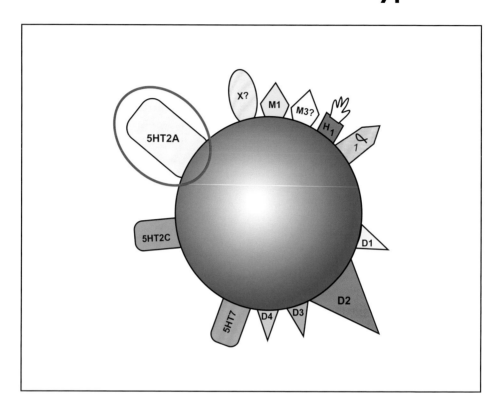

FIGURE 4.23. Originally developed as a conventional antipsychotic, especially at high doses, cyamemazine was later discovered to have 5HT2A antagonistic properties, especially at lower doses. This compound has high popularity in Europe, especially France, where it is used to treat anxiety associated with psychosis. Little information is available on its cardiometabolic and weight gain risks.

Cyamemazine: Tips and Pearls

	Dosing

Formulation:
25, 100 mg tablets; 40 mg/mL oral solution; 50 mg/5 mL injection

Dosage Range:
50-300 mg at bedtime (psychosis); 1-4 mg/kg/day (children 6 and older); 25-100 mg/day for injections

Approved For:
Not available in the USA

Pearls	
	Low dose has anxiolytic action and rarely causes motor side effects or prolactin elevation
	Used for severe behavioral disturbances in children and adolescents; oral solution preferred
	Not recommended during pregnancy or breast-feeding

Side effects I

Weight Gain

unusual | not unusual | common | problematic

Sedation

unusual | not unusual | **common** | problematic

 Rare neuroleptic malignant syndrome, rare seizures, rare agranulocytosis, jaundice, QTc prolongation

Side effects II

	Decreases effects of DA agonists; decreases BP in combo with epinephrine; increases effects of antihypertensive drugs
	Cardiovascular toxicity and orthostatic hypotension
	Use with caution in patients with renal impairments
	Use with caution in patients with hepatic impairments

FIGURE 4.24. Dosing and interaction information for cyamemazine.

Amisulpride

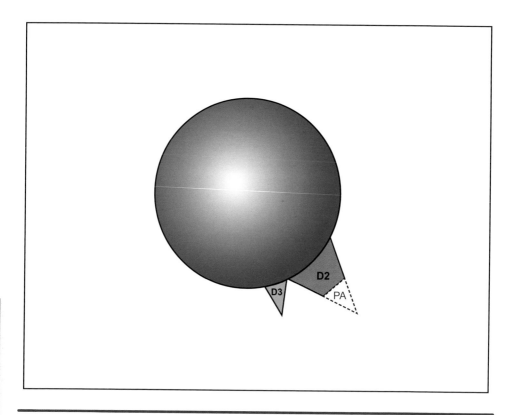

FIGURE 4.25. Amisulpride was developed in Europe before the concept of D2 partial agonism was fully accepted. It does not have any affinity at the 5HT2A receptor, and its side effect profile has not been fully investigated. It might lead to QTc prolongation and has been shown to induce prolactin elevation.

Amisulpride: Tips and Pearls

 Dosing

Formulation:
50, 100, 200 and 400 mg tablets;
100 mg/mL oral solution; IM
formulation

Dosage Range:
400-800 mg/day in 2 doses
(schizophrenia); 50-300 mg/day
(mainly negative symptoms)

Approved For:
Acute and chronic schizophrenia (in
Europe), not available in the USA

Pearls

 Efficacy in patients with
negative symptoms as low
doses are activating; increases
prolactin; could result in
amenorrhea

 Efficacy and safety not established under age 18

 Not recommended during
pregnancy or breast-feeding

Side effects I

Weight Gain

unusual   not unusual   common   problematic

Sedation

unusual   not unusual   common   problematic

 Rare neuroleptic ma-
lignant syndrome, rare
seizures, dose-depen-
dent QTc prolongation,
increased risk of death
in elderly, galactorrhea

Side effects II

 Increases effects of antihyper-
tensive drugs and decreases
effects of DA agonists; as it is
weakly metabolized, few drug
interactions exist

 Dose-dependent prolongation
of QTc interval

 Use with caution if renal insuf-
ficiency is present; drug can
accumulate, as it is eliminated
through the kidneys

 Use with caution in patients
with hepatic impairments

FIGURE 4.26. Dosing and interaction
information for amisulpride.

Sulpiride:
Conventional or Low-Dose Atypical?

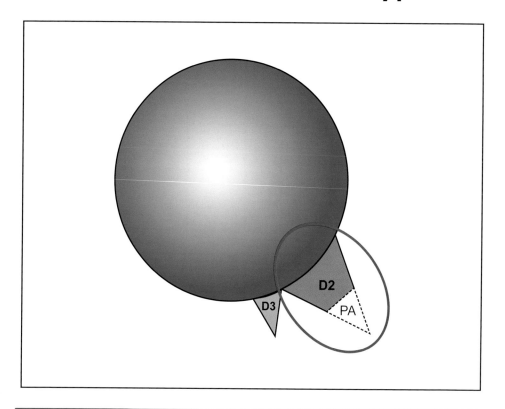

FIGURE 4.27. Sulpiride is structurally related to amisulpride. It too will lead to EPS and prolactin elevation at high doses, but it exhibits antidepressant actions and efficacy for negative symptoms at low doses.

Sulpiride: Tips and Pearls

	Dosing

Formulation:
200, 400 and 500 mg tablets; 50 and 100 mg/mL IM injections

Dosage Range:
400-800 mg/day in 2 doses (schizophrenia); 50-300 mg/day (mainly negative symptoms)

Approved For:
Not available in the USA

Pearls	
	Lower doses more effective for negative symptoms; lower doses are activating; higher doses are sedating
	Not recommended for use under age 15
	Potential risk should be weighed against potential benefit; drug found in breast milk

Side effects I

Weight Gain

unusual | not unusual | common | problematic

Sedation

unusual | not unusual | common | problematic

	Rare neuroleptic malignant syndrome, rare seizures, galactorrhea

Side effects II

	Increases effects of antihypertensive drugs and decreases effects of DA agonists; antacids reduce its absorption
	Use with caution in patients with cardiac impairments
	Use with caution if renal insufficiency is present; drug can accumulate, as it is eliminated through the kidneys
	Use with caution in patients with hepatic impairments

FIGURE 4.28. Dosing and interaction information for sulpiride.

Bifeprunox

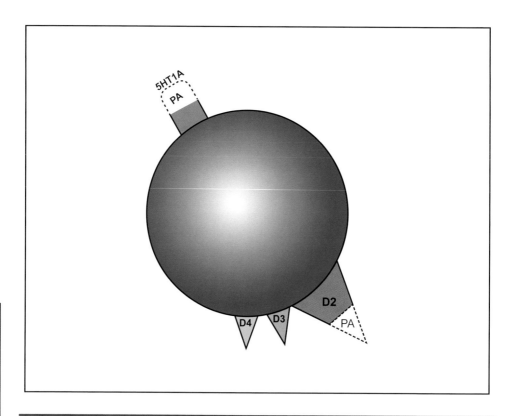

FIGURE 4.29. The D2 partial agonist bifeprunox is efficacious for positive symptoms in schizophrenia and for manic symptoms in bipolar disorder. Unlike other atypical antipsychotics it does not exhibit any 5HT2A antagonism. The D2 and 5HT1A partial agonism gives bifeprunox its pharmacological profile with low EPS and low hyperprolactinemia.

The absence of alpha 1, M1 and H1 properties ensures that bifeprunox does not have sedating properties. As it is close to a full agonist, it can induce vomiting and nausea, which can slow the dose titration and therefore the therapeutic action. The risks of weight gain and cardiometabolic side effects appear slim with bifeprunox. This agent is still in clinical testing and not yet available for use.

Iloperidone

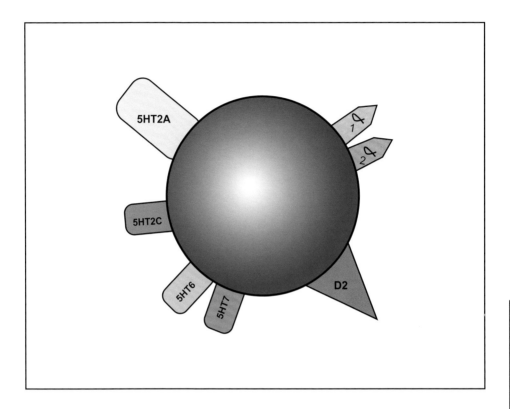

FIGURE 4.30. Iloperidone is one of the newer atypical antipsychotics with 5HT2A/D2 antagonistic properties. The doses used in clinical trials have been up to 32 mg/day, with an anticipated dose range of 12-24 mg/day given in divided doses. Similar side effects have been observed throughout the dosage range. Iloperidone exhibits dose-dependent QTc prolongation.

Early studies indicate iloperidone's efficacy in schizophrenia may be linked to certain pharmacogenetic markers. This agent is filed with the FDA as of this writing and not yet available for use.

Asenapine

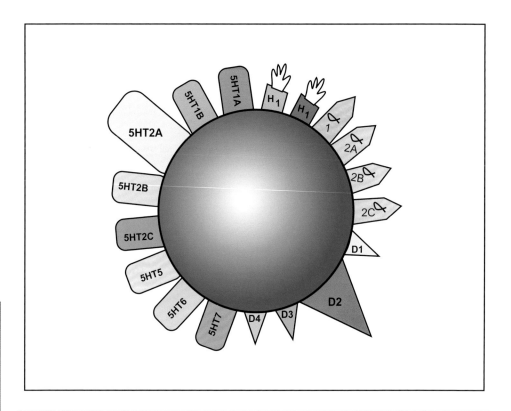

FIGURE 4.31. The newly developed atypical antipsychotic asenapine has a receptor profile even more complex than that of clozapine. It includes new properties such as actions at 5HT1B/2B receptors and alpha 2A, 2B and 2C properties. The relevance of actions at all these receptors is not yet known.

Asenapine has been developed as a sublingual formulation. Doses of 5 and 10 mg have been tested for mania and schizophrenia. Asenapine shows only mild metabolic risk and no prolactin elevation. This agent is filed with the FDA as of this writing and not yet available for use.

The Future of Antipsychotics

Table 4.1	
Compounds	**Properties and Notes**
Glycine agonists	Glycine, d-serine or its analogue d-cycloserine bind to the glycine site of the NMDA receptor, and could potentially stimulate the NMDA receptors enough to overcompensate for their hypothetical hypofunction; d-cycloserine is effective at treating negative and cognitive symptoms
GlyT1 inhibitors	Glycine transporter (GlyT1) inhibitors such as sarcosine block reuptake of glycine, thus increasing its synaptic availability. This could then lead to enhancement of NMDA neurotransmission and reversal of the hypofunctioning of NMDA receptors
mGluR agents	mGluR2/3 presynaptic receptor agonists could potentially decrease glutamate release; mGluR1 postsynaptic receptor agents can hypothetically modulate glutamate receptors and enhance postsynaptic NMDA-mediated neurotransmission
AMPA-kines	Positive allosteric modulators (PAMs) of this other glutamate receptor subtype, the AMPA receptor, can potentially enhance cognitive functioning
Sigma 1 agonists / antagonists	Sigma 1 receptors are linked to the psychotomimetic actions of PCP and regulate NMDA receptors. It is not yet known whether an agonist or antagonist would be best in schizophrenia; this is the "sigma enigma"
New 5HT agents	5HT2A-selective antagonists/inverse agonists, 5HT1A agonists/antagonists and 5HT2C agonists/antagonists are being investigated to improve cognitive effects and reduce side effects; 5HT6 antagonists might be beneficial by increasing brain-derived neurotrophic factor; 5HT7 antagonists could be beneficial for sleep and anxiety
New DA agents	D3 antagonists or partial agonists could potentially be useful to treat negative and cognitive symptoms and to alleviate stimulant abuse; D1 agonists and DA transporter inhibitors may be useful pro-cognitive agents
Acetylcholine-linked agents	Partial agonists at alpha-7-nicotinic cholinergic receptors may be pro-cognitive agents; varenicline, an alpha-4 beta-2 partial agonist, is approved for smoking cessation and could be beneficial in schizophrenia
Peptide-linked agents	Neurokinin antagonists have been tested, with unclear benefits; antagonists of neurotensin, which is colocalized with DA, are thought to reduce positive symptoms without inducing EPS. Cholecystokinin is also colocalized with DA, but no clear data on any compound are available

| Chapter 5

Schizophrenia Pharmacy and Switching Strategies

Figuring out how to treat schizophrenia in different patients can be challenging. Different "pharmacies" are presented in this chapter that can be useful in the search for an effective treatment plan. Practical switching strategies are also presented that will aid in properly changing medications in patients when different treatments are required.

Abbreviations Used in this Chapter	
AChEI	acetylcholinesterase inhibitor
BZ	benzodiazepine
D2	dopamine 2 antagonist
DPA	dopamine 2 partial antagonist
SDA	serotonin 2A and dopamine 2 antagonist
NRI	norepinephrine reuptake inhibitor
SSRI	selective serotonin reuptake inhibitor

The Puzzle of Schizophrenia

FIGURE 5.1. Schizophrenia is an aggregation of different symptoms, including positive, negative, aggressive, affective, and cognitive ones. One medication may not treat all of a patient's symptoms effectively.

Likewise, a patient might not present with the full panoply of symptoms and might thus require specific treatment. Thus it is beneficial to know which medications are more efficacious at treating different symptom dimensions.

Treating Positive Symptoms

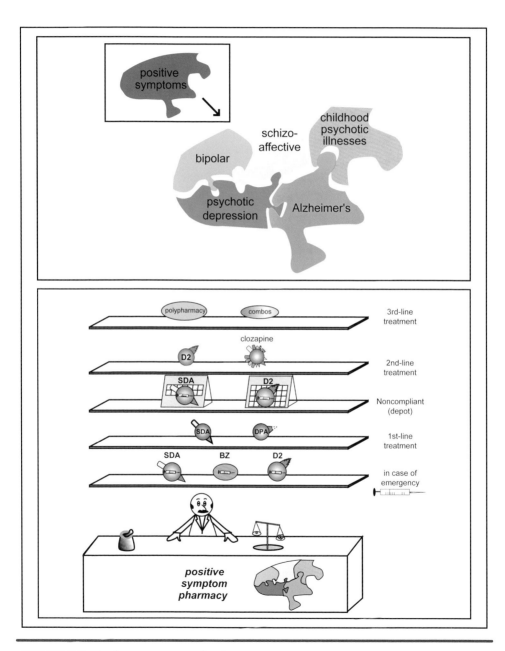

FIGURE 5.2. The best treatments for the positive symptoms of schizophrenia.

Treating Negative Symptoms

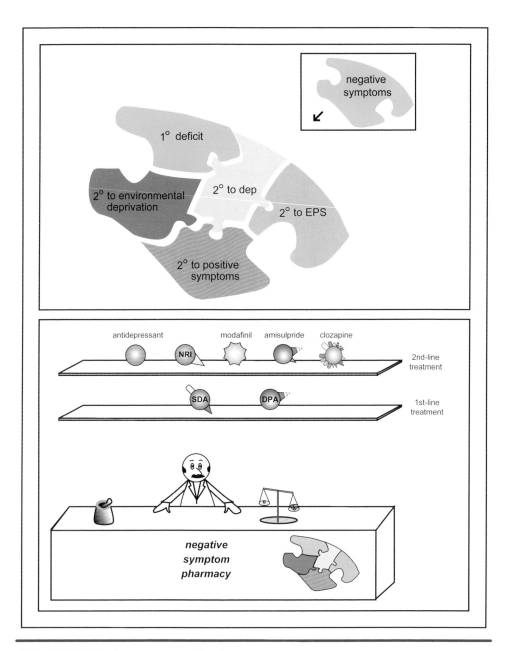

FIGURE 5.3. The best treatments for the negative symptoms of schizophrenia.

Treating Cognitive Symptoms

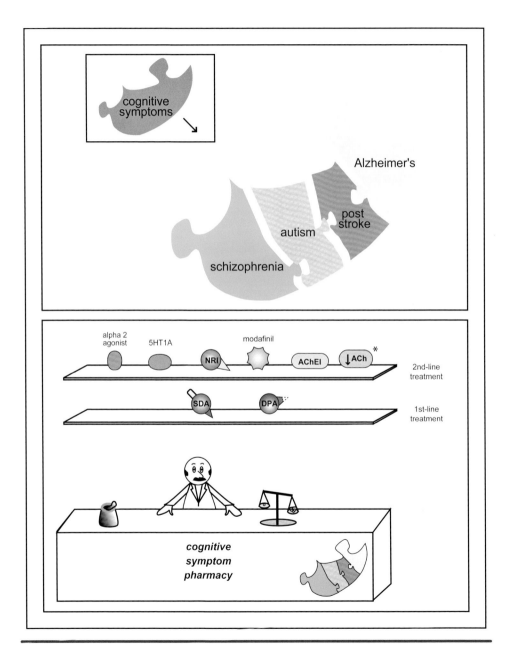

FIGURE 5.4. The best treatments for the cognitive symptoms of schizophrenia.

*↓ACh = decrease anticholinergics

Treating Aggressive Symptoms

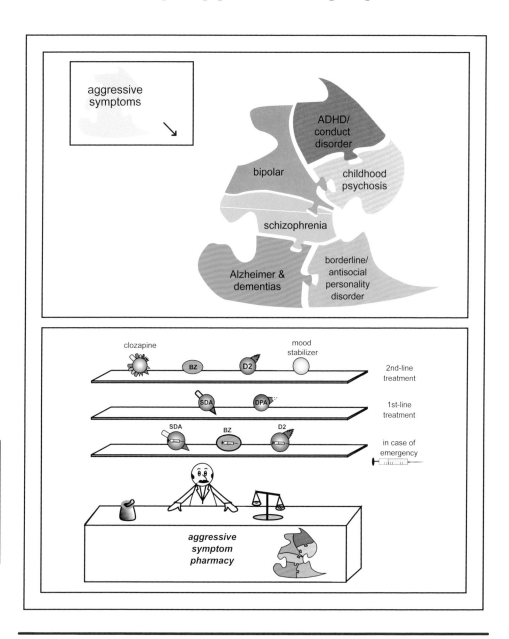

FIGURE 5.5. The best treatments for the aggressive symptoms of schizophrenia.

Treating Affective Symptoms

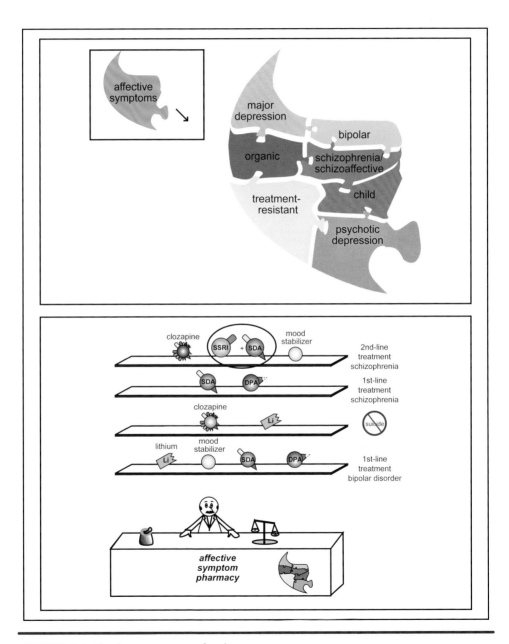

FIGURE 5.6. The best treatments for the affective symptoms of schizophrenia.

Treating Metabolic Issues

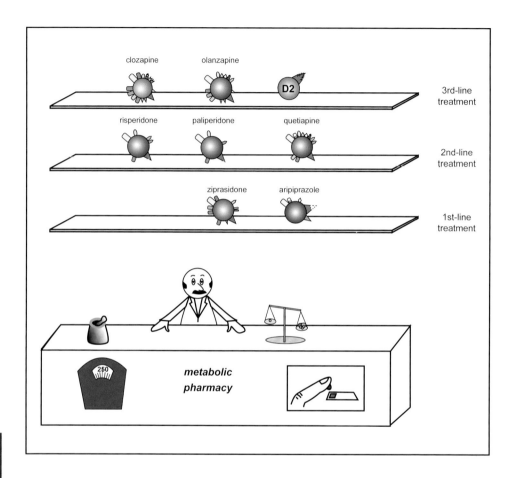

FIGURE 5.7. Aripiprazole and ziprasidone appear to have lower risks for cardiometabolic problems and weight gain, and therefore represent the first-line treatment in the metabolic pharmacy. Risperidone, paliperidone and quetiapine are second-line treatment options as they carry an intermediate risk to gain weight and develop cardiometabolic side effects.

Olanzapine and clozapine have the highest risk of weight gain and therefore cardiometabolic disease, and should only be used as third-line treatment. Some of the conventional antipsychotics might actually carry less risk of cardiometabolic side effects, but more research is required.

Treating Sedation

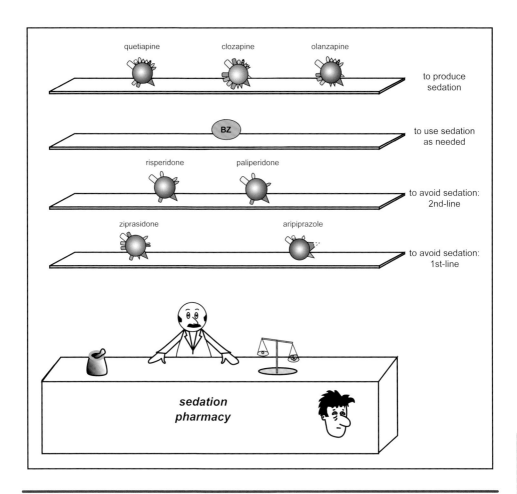

FIGURE 5.8. Ziprasidone and aripiprazole are the antipsychotics with the least tendency to induce sedation. Risperidone and paliperidone have been known to induce sedation in some patients, but not in others.

If sedation is wanted, then compounds such as quetiapine, clozapine, or olanzapine should be used. Augmentation with a benzodiazepine can also lead to sedation.

How Not to Switch Antipsychotics

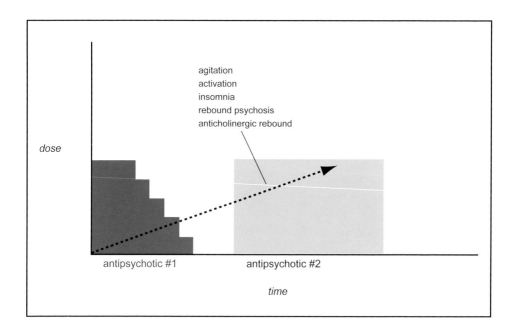

FIGURE 5.9. There are strategies for switching antipsychotics and strategies to avoid in order to prevent rebound psychosis, aggravation of side effects, or withdrawal symptoms.

Generally, it is preferable to (1) not rush the discontinuation of the first antipsychotic, (2) not allow gaps between two antipsychotic treatments, and (3) not start the second antipsychotic at full dose.

Switching from One Sedating Antipsychotic to Another

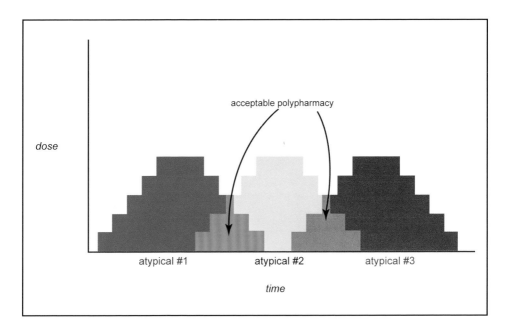

FIGURE 5.10. Cross-titration is usually advised when switching from one sedating antipsychotic to another. As the first antipsychotic is slowly tapered off, the second antipsychotic is slowly added on. This can be done over a few days or a few weeks. Even though the patient will be simultaneously taking two medications for a short period of time, this is acceptable as it can decrease side effects and the risk of rebound symptoms, and it can hasten the successful transition to the second drug.

Getting Trapped in Cross-Titration

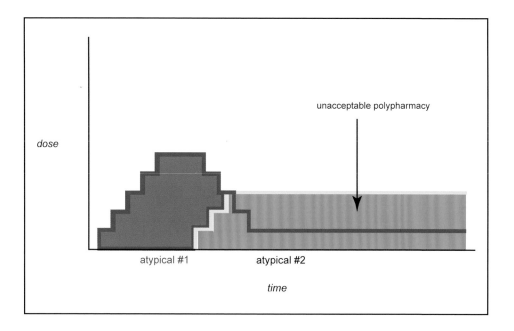

FIGURE 5.11. When initiating cross-titration, it is imperative to not forget to taper the first drug. Patients may improve in the middle of a cross-titration, but this should not be the reason to stop the process. An unfinished cross-titration will lead to polypharmacy where the patient takes two drugs indefinitely.

While polypharmacy is sometimes a necessity in hard-to-treat cases, an adequate monotherapy trial of a second drug should be the first option.

Use of Benzodiazepines to "Lead In" or "Top Up" Nonsedating Antipsychotics

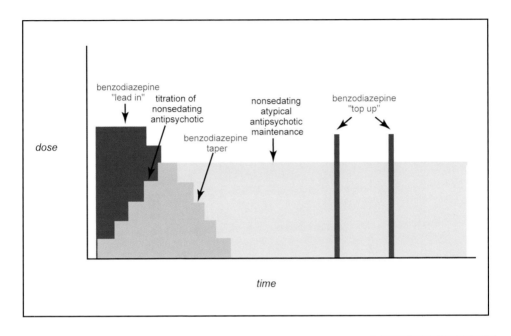

FIGURE 5.12. Benzodiazepines have been useful to either "lead in" or "top up" a nonsedating antipsychotic. When patients are agitated, it may be beneficial to augment with a benzodiazepine just for a short time when the nonsedating antipsychotic is initiated. Thus the benzodiazepine is used as a "lead in" to the nonsedating antipsychotic. Once the nonsedating antipsychotic has been titrated to its full dose, then the benzodiazepine can be slowly tapered. Additionally, during the maintenance phase of the antipsychotic it can be helpful to use a benzodiazepine as a "top up" when needed by the patient.

Switching from a Sedating to a Nonsedating Antipsychotic

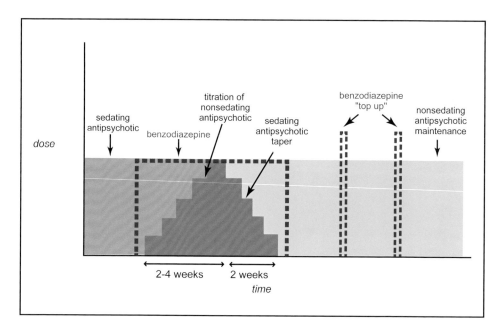

FIGURE 5.13. Switching from a sedating to a nonsedating antipsychotic can be problematic. One method for doing this is shown above. First a benzodiazepine is added, and then the nonsedating antipsychotic is titrated to its optimal therapeutic dose, while the sedating antipsychotic is still given at full dose. At this point the sedating antipsychotic is slowly tapered, while keeping the benzodiazepine present. When the patient is stable, the benzodiazepine can be tapered or stopped. Occasionally the benzodiazepine can be used to "top up" the patient and treat agitation or insomnia.

This switching strategy may be best for patients who are switching due to lack of adequate control of symptoms by their sedating antipsychotic. For those who are switching due to intolerability, the temporary polypharmacy of three agents may lead to side effects.

Switching from an SDA to a DPA: Not Too Fast

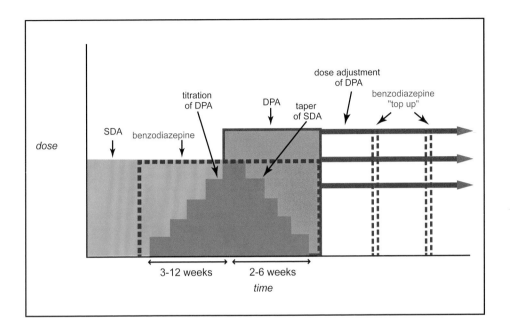

FIGURE 5.14. The emergence of psychosis, agitation, and insomnia can potentially burden the switch from a 5HT2A/D2 antagonist (SDA) to a D2 partial agonist (DPA). It may be best to initially add the second antipsychotic gradually while keeping the first one at full dose, and to keep both medications on board for a few weeks. It may also be beneficial to add a benzodiazepine short-term.

As soon as the patient is stable, the benzodiazepine can be tapered or stopped. Occasionally the benzodiazepine can be used to "top up" the patient and treat agitation or insomnia. When switching to a partial D2 agonist, it is important to give the receptors time to adjust their sensitivity, and thus the dose of the DPA may need to be adjusted in order to reach full therapeutic potential.

When Several Antipsychotic Monotherapies Fail

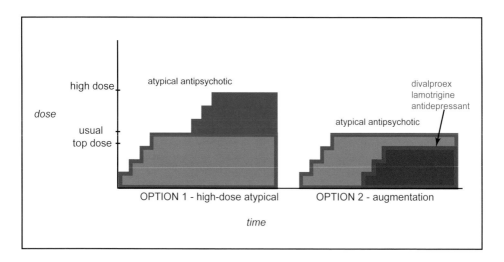

FIGURE 5.15. When a monotherapy with an atypical antipsychotic fails, the psychopharmacologist has few options.

Left: A high dose of the atypical antipsychotic can be used; however at high doses some side effects might appear that are normally not related to atypical antipsychotics.

Right: Augmentation with a mood stabilizer such as divalproex or lamotrigine or with an antidepressant could transform a previously ineffective atypical antipsychotic monotherapy into an efficacious drug cocktail.

When All Else Fails

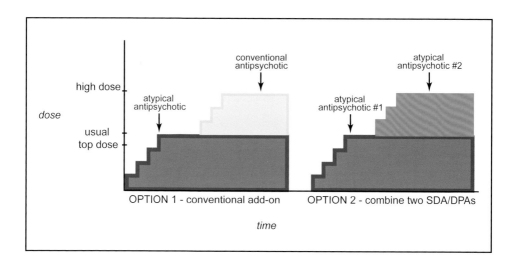

FIGURE 5.16. When pushing the dose of an atypical antipsychotic or augmenting it with other drugs still fails, it might be necessary to combine two antipsychotics. A conventional antipsychotic (left), or an atypical antipsychotic such as an SDA or DPA (right) can be added to the first atypical drug.

While antipsychotic polypharmacy is frequently practiced, it has not been well-studied and should only be used when every other approach has failed.

Summary

- The underlying pathophysiology of schizophrenia remains to be fully elucidated.

- Dopamine, glutamate and serotonin are three of the most important neurotransmitter systems involved in schizophrenia and in the mechanism of action of conventional and atypical antipsychotics.

- Each antipsychotic has a unique receptor profile, important in the alleviation of symptoms and induction of side effects.

- Atypical antipsychotics can have cardiometabolic risks, and thus patients need to be monitored when treatment is initiated.

- Today's psychopharmacologist has many choices when it comes to choosing an antipsychotic and can individualize treatment with the goals of maximizing treatment and minimizing side effects.

- It is necessary for psychopharmacologists to understand the art of switching between different antipsychotics, as patients will most likely have to try different medications in order to reach an optimal treatment plan.

Abbreviations and Symbols

5HT	serotonin	Li	lithium
A	amygdala	mGluR	metabotropic glutamate receptor
ACh	acetylcholine		
AChEI	acetylcholinesterase inhibitor	NA	nucleus accumbens
		NE	norepinephrine
AMPA	alpha-amino-3-hydroxy-5-methyl-4-isoxazoleproprionic acid	NMDA	N-methyl-*d*-aspartate
		NRI	norepinephrine reuptake inhibitor
BP	blood pressure	NT	brainstem neurotransmitter center
BF	basal forebrain		
BMI	body mass index	PA	partial agonist
BZ	benzodiazepine	PAM	positive allosteric modulator
C	cerebellum	PCP	phencyclidine
CYP450	cytochrome P450 system	PFC	prefrontal cortex
DA	dopamine	S	striatum
DKA	diabetic ketoacidosis	SC	spinal cord
DLPFC	dorsolateral prefrontal cortex	SDA	serotonin 2A and dopamine 2 antagonist
DPA	dopamine 2 partial agonist	SPA	serotonin 1A partial agonist
EPS	extrapyramidal side effects	SSRI	selective serotonin reuptake inhibitor
GABA	gamma-aminobutyric acid		
glu	glucose	T	thalamus
GLU	glutamate	TG	triglycerides
GlyT1	glycine transporter	VMPFC	ventromedial prefrontal cortex
H	hippocampus		
HA	histamine	VTA	ventral tegmental area
Hy	hypothalamus		

	Life-threatening or Dangerous Side Effects		Drug Interactions
	Tips and Pearls		Cardiac Impairment
	Children and Adolescents		Renal Impairment
	Pregnancy		Hepatic Impairment

Suggested Readings

Abbatecola AM, Rizzo MR, Barbieri M, Grella R, Arciello A, Laieta MT et al. Post prandial plasma glucose excursions and cognitive functioning in aged type 2 diabetics. Neurology 2006;67(7):235–40.

Agid O, Mamo D, Ginovart N, Vitcu I, Wilson AA, Zipursky RB et al. Striatal vs. extrastriatal dopamine D2 receptors in antipsychotic response – a double-blind pet study in schizophrenia. Neuropsychopharmacology 2007;32:1209–15.

Alphs LD, Summerfelt A, Lann H, Muller RJ. The negative symptom assessment: a new instrument to assess negative symptoms of schizophrenia. Psychopharmacol Bull1989;25(2):159–63.

Artaloytia JF, Arango C, Lahti A, Sanz J, Pascual A, Cubero P et al. Negative signs and symptoms secondary to antipsychotics: a double-blind, randomized trial of a single dose of placebo, haloperidol, and risperidone in healthy volunteers. Am J Psychiatry 2006;163(3):488–93.

Atmaca M, Kuloglu M, Tezcan E, Ustundag B. Serum leptin and triglyceride levels in patients on treatment with atypical antipsychotics. J Clin Psychiatry 2003;64(5):598–604.

Bai YM, Lin CC, Chen JY, Lin CY, Su TP, Chou P. Association of initial antipsychotic response to clozapine and long-term weight gain. Am J Psychiatry 2006;163:1276–9.

Bardin L, Kleven MS, Barret-Grevoz C, Depoortere R, Newman-Tancredi A. Antipsychotic-like vs. cataleptogenic actions in mice of novel antipsychotics having D2 antagonist and 5-HT1A agonist properties. Neuropsychopharmacology 2006;31:1869–79.

Bennett S, Gronier B. Modulation of striatal dopamine release in vitro by agonists of the glycineB site of NMDA receptors: interaction with antipsychotics. Eur J Pharmacol 2005;527:52–9.

Bota RG, Sagduyu K, Munro JS. Factors associated with the prodromal progression of schizophrenia that influence the course of the illness. CNS Spectr 2005;10(12):937–42.

Cannon TD, Glahn DC, Kim J, Van Erp TGH, Karlsgodt K, Cohen MS et al. Dorsolateral prefrontal cortex activity during maintenance and manipulation of information in working memory in patients with schizophrenia. Arch Gen Psychiatry 2005;62:1071–80.

Chiu CC, Chen KP, Liu HC, Lu ML. The early effect of olanzapine and risperidone on insulin secretion in atypical-naive schizophrenic patients. J Clin Psychopharmacol 2006;26(5):504–7.

Citrome L, Jaffe A, Levine J, Martello D. Incidence, prevalence and surveillance for diabetes in New York State psychiatric hospitals, 1997–2004. Psychiatr Serv 2006;57(8)1132–9.

Citrome L, Macher JP, Salazar DE, Mallikaarjun S, Boulton DW. Pharmacokinetics of aripiprazole and concomitant carbamazepine. J Clin Psychopharmacol 2007;27(3):279–83.

Coyle JT, Tsai G. The NMDA receptor glycine modulatory site: a therapeutic target for improving cognition and reducing negative symptoms in schizophrenia. Psychopharmacology 2004;174:32–8.

Coyle JT, Tsai G, Goff D. Converging evidence of NMDA receptor hypofunction in the pathophysiology of schizophrenia. Ann N Y Acad Sci 2003;1003:318–27.

Coyle JT. Glutamate and schizophrenia: beyond the dopamine hypothesis. Cell Mol Neurobiol 2006;26(4–6):365–84.

De Bartolomeis A, Fiore G, Iasevoli F. Dopamine-glutamate interaction and antipsychotics mechanism of action: implication for new pharmacological strategies in psychosis. Curr Pharm Design 2005;11:3561–94.

DiForti M, Lappin JM, Murray RM. Risk factors for schizophrenia – all roads lead to dopamine. Eur Neuropsychopharmacol 2007;17:S101–7.

Emsley R, Rabinowitz J, Medori R. Time course for antipsychotic treatment response in first-episode schizophrenia. Am J Psychiatry 2006;163:743–5.

Essock SM, Covell NH, Davis SM, Stroup TS, Rosenheck RA, Lieberman JA. Effectiveness of switching antipsychotic medications. Am J Psychiatry 2006;163(12):2090–5.

Fenton WS, Chavez MR. Medication-induced weight gain and dyslipidemia in patients with schizophrenia. Am J Psychiatry 2006;163:1697–1704.

Glenthoj BY, Mackeprang T, Svarer C, Rasmussen H, Pinborg LH, Friberg L et al. Frontal dopamine D2/3 receptor binding in drug naive first-episode schizophrenia patients correlates with positive psychotic symptoms and gender. Biol Psychiatry 2006;60:621–9.

Green MF, Marder SR, Glynn SM, McGurk SR, Wirshing WC, Wirshing DA et al. The neurocognitive effects of low-dose haloperidol: a two-year comparison with risperidone. Biol Psychiatry 2002;51:972–8.

Henderson DC, Cagliero E, Copeland PM, Louie PM, Borba CP, Fan X et al. Elevated hemoglobin A1c as a possible indicator of diabetes mellitus and diabetic ketoacidosis in schizophrenia patients receiving atypical antipsychotics. J Clin Psychiatry 2007;68:533–41.

Heresco-Levy U, Bar G, Levin R, Ermilov M, Ebstein RP, Javitt DC. High glycine levels are associated with prepulse inhibition deficits in chronic schizophrenia patients. Schizophr Res 2007;91(1–3):14–21.

Heresco-Levy U, Javitt DC, Ebstein R, Vass Ag, Lichtenbwerg P, Bar G et al. D-serine efficacy as add-on pharmacotherapy to risperidone and olanzapine for treatment-refractory schizophrenia. Biol Psychiatry 2005;57:577–85.

Houseknecht KL, Robertson AS, Zavadoski W, Gibbs EM, Johnson DE, Rollema H. Acute effects of atypical antipsychotics on whole-body insulin resistance in rats: implications for adverse metabolic effects. Neuropsychopharmacology 2007;32:289–97.

Hoyer D, Hannon JP, Martin GR. Molecular, pharmacological and functional diversity of 5-HT receptors. Pharmacol Biochem Behav 2002;71:533–54.

Ingelman-Sundberg M. Pharmacogenetics of cytochrome P450 and its applications in drug therapy: the past, present and future. Trends in Pharmacol Sci 2004;25(4):193–200.

Javitt DC. Is the glycine site half saturated or half unsaturated? Effects of glutamatergic drugs in schizophrenia patients. Curr Opin Psychiatry 2006;19:151–7.

Javitt DC, Balla A, Burch S, Suckow R, Xie S, Sershen H. Reversal of phencyclidine-induced dopaminergic dysregulation by N-methyl-d-aspartate receptor/glycine-site agonists. Neuropsychopharmacology 2004;(29):300–7.

Jindal RD, Keshavan S. Critical role of M3 muscarinic receptor in insulin secretion. J Clin Psychopharmacol 2006;26(5):449–50.

Johnson DE, Yamazaki H, Ward KM, Schmidt AW, Lebel WS, Treadway JL et al. Inhibitory effects of antipsychotics on carbachol-enhanced insulin secretion from perifused rat islets. Diabetes 2005;54:1552–8.

Jones PB, Barnes TRE, Davies L, Dunn G, Lloyd H, Hayhurst KP, Murray RM et al. Randomized controlled trial of the effect on quality of life of second- vs. first-generation antipsychotic drugs in schizophrenia. Arch Gen Psychiatry 2006;63:1079–87.

Kahn RS, Schulz SC, Palazov VD, Reyes EB, Brecher M, Svensson O et al. Efficacy and tolerability of once daily extended release quetiapine fumarate in acute schizophrenia: a randomized, double blind, placebo controlled study. J Clin Psychiatry 2007;68(6):832–42.

Kalkman HO, Feuerbach D, Lotscher E, Schoeffter P. Functional characterization of the novel antipsychotic iloperidone at human D2, D3, Alpha2c, 5-HT6 and 5-HT1A receptors. Life Sci 2003;73:1151–9.

Kapur S, Lecrubier Y. editors. Dopamine in the pathophysiology and treatment of schizophrenia. London, Martin Dunitz; 2003.

Kapur S. Psychosis as a state of aberrant salience: a framework linking biology, phenomenology, and pharmacology in schizophrenia. Am J Psychiatry 2003;160(1):13–23.

Keefe RS, Bilder RM, Davis SM, Harvey PD, Palmer BW, Gold JM et al.

Neurocognitive effects of antipsychotic medications in patients with chronic schizophrenia in the CATIE trial. Arch Gen Psychiatry 2007;64:633–47.

Keefe RS, Bilder RM, Harvey PD, Davis SM, Palmer BW, Gold JM et al. Baseline neurocognitive deficits in the CATIE schizophrenia trial. Neuropsychopharmacology 2006;31:2033–46.

Keefe RS, Seidman LJ, Christensen BK, Harner RM, Sharma T, Sitskoorn MM et al. Long-term neurocognitive effects of olanzapine or low-dose haloperidol in first episode psychosis. Biol Psychiatry 2006;59:97–105.

Kern RS, Green MF, Cornblatt BA, Owen JR, McQuade RD, Carson WH et al. The neurocognitive effects of aripiprazole: an open label comparison with olanzapine. Psychopharmacology 2006;187:312–20.

Kessler RM, Ansari MS, Riccardi P, Li R, Jayathilake K, Dawant B et al. Occupancy of striatal and extrastriatal dopamine D2 receptors by clozapine and quetiapine. Neuropsychopharmacology 2006;31:1991–2001.

Kessler RM, Ansari MS, Riccardi P, Li R, Jyathilake K, Dawant B et al. Occupancy of striatal and extrastriatal dopamine D2/D3 receptors by olanzapine and haloperidol. Neuropsychopharmacology 2005;30:2283–9.

Lambert BL, Cunningham FE, Miller DR, Dalack GW, Hur K. Diabetes risk associated with use of olanzapine, quetiapine, and risperidone in Veterans Health Administration patients with schizophrenia. Am J Epidemiol 2006;164:672–81.

Lamberti JS, Olson D, Crilly JF, Olivares T, Williams GC, Tu X et al. Prevalence of the metabolic syndrome among patients receiving clozapine. Am J Psychiatry 2006;163:1273–6.

Lane HY, Chang YC, Liu YC, Chiu CC, Tsai GE. Sarcosine or D-Serine add-on treatment for acute exacerbation of schizophrenia. Arch Gen Psychiatry 2005;62:1196–1204.

Lane HY, Huang CL, Wu PL, Liu YC, Chang YC, Lin PY et al. Glycine Transporter 1 inhibitor, N-methylglycine (sarcosine), added to clozapine for the treatment of schizophrenia. Biol Psychiatry 2006;60:645–9.

Lawler CP, Prioleau C, Lewis MM, Mak C, Jiang D, Schetz JA et al. Interactions of the novel antipsychotic aripiprazole (OPC-14597) with dopamine and serotonin receptor su types. Neuropsychopharmacology 1999;20(6):612–27.

Lencz T, Smith CW, McLaughlin D, Auther A, Nakayama E, Hovey L et al. Generalized and specific neurocognitive deficits in prodromal schizophrenia. Biol Psychiatry 2006;59:863–71.

Leucht S, Busch R, Math D, Kissling W, Kane JM. Early prediction of antipsychotic nonresponse among patients with schizophrenia. J Clin Psychiatry 2007;68(3):352–60.

Lieberman JA, Stroup TS, McEvoy JP, Swartz MS, Rosenheck RA, Perkins DO, et al. Effectiveness of antipsychotic drugs in patients with chronic schizophernia. N Engl J Med 2005;353(12):1209-23.

Lieberman JA, Tollefson GD, Charles C, Zipursky R, Sharma T, Kahn RS et al. Antipsychotic drug effects on brain morphology in first episode psychosis. Arch

Gen Psychiatry 2005;62:361–70.

Lindenmayer JP, Khan A, Iskander A, Abad MT, Parker B. A randomized controlled trial of olanzapine versus haloperidol in the treatment of primary negative symptoms and neurocognitive deficits in schizophrenia. J Clin Psychiatry 2007;68(3):368–79.

Lipkovich I, Citrome L, Perlis R, Deberdt W, Jouston JP, Ahl J et al. Early predictors of substantial weight gain in bipolar patients treated with olanzapine. J Clin Psychopharmocol 2006;26(3):316–20.

Lynch G, Gall CM. Ampakines and the threefold path to cognitive enhancement. Trends Neurosci 2006;29:10.

McCreary AD, Glennon JC, Ashby Jr R, Meltzer HY, Li Z, Reinders JH et al. SLV313 (1-(2,3 dihydro-benzo[1,4] dioxin-5-yl)-4-[5-(4-fluoro-phenyl)-Pyridin-3-ylmethyl]-piperazine monohydrochloride): a novel dopamine D2 receptor Antagonist and 5-HT1A receptor agonist potential antipsychotic drug. Neuropsychopharmacology 2007;32:78–94.

McEvoy JP, Lieberman JA, Sroup TS, Davis SM, Meltzer HY, Rosenheck RA et al. Effectiveness of clozapine versus olanzapine, quetiapine, and risperidone in patients with chronic schizophrenia who did not respond to prior atypical antipsychotic treatment. Am J Psychiatry 2006;163:600–10.

McGlashan TH, Zipursky RB, Perkins D, Addington J, Miller T, Woods SW et al. Randomized, double-blind trial of olanzapine versus placebo in patients prodromally symptomatic for psychosis. Am J Psychiatry 2006;163:790–9.

McLaughlin T, Abbasi F, Cheal K, Chu J, Lamendola C, Reaven G. Use of metabolic markers to identify overweight individuals who are insulin resistant. Ann Intern Med 2003;139:802–9.

Millan MJ. N-Methyl-d-aspartate receptors as a target for improved antipsychotic agents: novel insights and clinical perspectives. Psychopharmacology 2005;179:30–53.

Mizrahi R, Rusjan P, Agid O, Graff A, Mamo DC, Zipursky RB et al. Adverse subjective experience with antipsychotics and its relationship to striatal and extrastriatal D2 receptors: a PET study in schizophrenia. Am J Psychiatry 2007;164:630–7.

Murphy BP, Chung YC, Park TW, McGorry PD. Pharmacological treatment of primary negative symptoms in schizophrenia: a systematic review. Schizophr Res 2006;88:5–25.

Natesan S, Reckless GE, Barlow KBL, Nobrega JN, Kapur S. Evaluation of N-desmethylclozapine as a potential antipsychotic – preclinical studies. Neuropsychopharmacology 2007;32:1540–9.

Natesan S, Reckless GE, Nobrega JN, Fletcher PJ, Kapur S. Dissociation between in vivo occupancy and functional antagonism of dopamine D2 receptors: comparing aripiprazole to other antipsychotics in animal models. Neuropsychopharmacology 2006;31:1854–63.

Newman-Tancredi A, Assie MB, Leduc N, Ormiere AM, Danty N, Cosi C. Novel antipsychotics activate recombinant human and native rat serotonin 5-HT1A receptors: affinity, efficacy and potential implications for treatment of schizophrenia. Int J Neuropsychopharmacol 2005;8:341–56.

Olfson M, Blanco C, Liu L, Moreno C, Laje G. National trends in the outpatient treatment of children and adolescents with antipsychotic drugs. Arch Gen Psychiatry 2006;63:679–85.

Olfson M, Marcus SC, Corey-Lisle P, Tuomari AV, Hines P, L'Italien GJ. Hyperlipidemia following treatment with antipsychotic medications. Am J Psychiatry 2006;163:1821–5.

Olincy A, Harris JG, Johnson LL, Pender V, Kongs S, Allensworth D et al. Proof-of-concept trial of an alpha 7 nicotinic agonist in schizophrenia. Arch Gen Psychiatry 2006;63:630–8.

Osborn DPJ, Levy G, Nazareth I, Petersen I, Islam A, King MB. Relative risk of cardiovascular and cancer mortality in people with severe mental illness from the United Kingdom's general practice research database. Arch Gen Psychiatry 2007;64:242–9.

Pierre JM, Peloian JH, Wirshing DA,Wirshing WC, Marder SR. A randomized, double-blind, placebo-controlled trial of modafinil for negative symptoms in schizophrenia. J Clin Psychiatry 2007;68(5):705–10.

Polsky D, Doshi JA, Bauer MS, Glick HA. Clinical trial-based cost effectiveness analyses of antipsychotic use. Am J Psychiatry 2006;163(12):2047–56.

Reaven G. The metabolic syndrome or the insulin resistance syndrome: different names, different concepts, and different goals. Endocrinol Metab Clin North Am 2004;33:283–303.

Reist C, Mintz J, Albers LJ, Jamas MM, Szabo S, Ozdemir V. Second-generation antipsychotic exposure and metabolic-related disorders in patients with schizophrenia. J Clin Psychopharmacol 2007;27:46–51.

Remington G, Mamo D, Labelle A, Reiss J, Shammi C, Mannaert E et al. A PET study evaluating dopamineD2 receptor occupancy for long-acting injectable risperidone. Am J Psychiatry 2006;163(3):396–401.

Reyes M, Buitelaar J, Toren P, Augustyns I, Eerdekens M. A randomized, double-blind, placebo-controlled study of risperidone maintenance treatment in children and adolescents with disruptive behavior disorders. Am J Psychiatry 2006;163:402–10.

Reynolds GP, Yao Z, Zhang XB, Sun J, Zhang ZJ. Pharmacogenetics of treatment in first-episode schizophrenia: D3 and 5-HT2C receptor polymorphisms separately associate with positive and negative symptom response. Eur Neuropsychopharmacol 2004;15:143–51.

Rosenheck RA, Leslie DL, Sindelar J, Miller EA, Lin H, Stroup TS et al. Cost-effectiveness of second generation antipsychotics and perphenazine in a randomized trial of treatment for chronic schizophrenia. Am J Psychiatry 2006;163(12):2080–9.

Sarter M. Preclinical research into cognition enhancers. Trends Pharmacol Sci

2006;27:11.

Sepehry AA, Potvin S, Elie R, Stip E. Selective serotonin reuptake inhibitor (SSRI) add-on therapy for the negative symptoms of schizophrenia: a meta-analysis. J Clin Psychiatry 2007;68(4):604–10.

Shayegan DK, Stahl SM. Emotion processing, the amygdala, and outcome in schizophrenia. Prog Neuropsychopharmacol Biol Psychiatry 2005;29:840–5.

Simonson GD, Kendall DM. Diagnosis of insulin resistance and associated syndromes: the spectrum from the metabolic syndrome to type 2 diabetes mellitus. Coron Artery Dis 2005;16:465–72.

Smid P, Coolen HKAC, Keizer HG, van Hes R, de Moes JP, den Hartog AP et al. Synthesis, structure-activity relationships, and biological properties of 1-heteroaryl-4-[Ω-(1H-indol-3-yl) alkyl]piperazines, novel potential antipsychotics combining potent dopamine D2 receptor antagonism with potent serotonin reuptake inhibition. J Med Chem 2005;48:6855–69.

Spurling RD, Lamberti JS, Olsen D, Tu X, Tang W. Changes in metabolic parameters with switching to aripiprazole from another second-generation antipsychotic: a retrospective chart review. J Clin Psychiatry 2007;68(3):406–9.

Stahl SM. Prophylactic antipsychotics: do they keep you from catching schizophrenia? J Clin Psychiatry 2004;65(11):1445–6.

Stahl SM. Stahl's Essential Psychopharmacology, 3rd Edition, Cambridge University Press, N.Y., 2008.

Stahl SM. Stahl's Essential Psychopharmacology: Prescriber's Guide, 2nd Edition, Cambridge University Press, N.Y., 2006.

Stroup TS, Lieberman JA, McEvoy JP, Swartz MS, Davis SM, Capuano GA et al. Effectiveness of olanzapine, quetiapine, and risperidone in patients with chronic schizophrenia after discontinuing perphenazine: a CATIE study. Am J Psychiatry 2007;164:415–27.

Takahashi H, Higuchi M, Suhara T. The role of extrastriatal dopamine D2 receptors in schizophrenia. Biol Psychiatry 2006;59:919–28.

Talkowski ME, Mansour H, Chowdari KV, Wood J, Butler A, Varma PG et al. Novel, replicated associations between dopamine D3 receptor gene polymorphisms and schizophrenia in two independent samples. Biol Psychiatry 2006;60:570–7.

Tarazi FI, Baldessarini RJ, Kula NS, Zhang K. Long-term effects of olanzapine, risperidone, and quetiapine on ionotropic glutamate receptor types: implications for antipsychotic drug treatment. J Pharmacol Exp Ther 2003;306(3):1145–51.

Tenback DE, van Harten PN, Sloof CJ, van Os J. Evidence that early extrapyramidal symptoms predict later tardive dyskinesia: a prospective analysis of 10,000 patients in the European schizophrenia outpatient health outcomes (SOHO) study. Am J Psychiatry 2006;163:1438–40.

Tran-Johnson TK, Sack DA, Marcus RN, Auby P, McQuade RD, Oren DA. Efficacy and safety of intramuscular aripiprazole in patients with acute agitation: a randomized, double-blind, placebo-controlled trial. J Clin Psychiatry 2007;68(1):111–9.

Tsai G, Lane HY, Chong MY, Lange N. Glycine transporter 1 inhibitor, N-methylglycine (sarcosine), added to antipsychotics for the treatment of schizophrenia. Biol Psychiatry 2004;55:452–6.

Vestri HS, Maianu L, Moellering DR, Garvey WT. Atypical antipsychotic drugs directly impair insulin action in adipocytes: effects on glucose transport, lipogenesis, and antilipolysis. Neuropsychopharmacology 2007;32:765–72.

Vidalis AA. Psychopharmacology issues in pregnancy and lactation. Thessasloniki, Greece, Contemporary Editions; 2006.

Weissman EM, Zhu CW, Schooler NR, Goetz RR, Essock SM. Lipid monitoring in patients with schizophrenia prescribed second generation antipsychotics. J Clin Psychiatry 2006;67(9):1323–6.

Wezenberg E, Verkes RJ, Ruigt GSF, Hulstijn W, Sabbe BGC. Acute effects of the ampakine farampator on memory and information processing in healthy elderly volunteers. Neuropsychopharmacology 2007;32:1272–83.

Yaeger D, Smith HG, Altshuler LL. Atypical antipsychotics in the treatment of schizophrenia during pregnancy and the postpartum. Am J Psychiatry 2006;163(12):2064–70.

Zhang M, Ballard ME, Kohlhaas KL, Browmna KE, Jongen-Relo AL, Unger LV et al. Effect of dopamine D3 antagonists on PPI in DBA/2J mice or PPI deficit induced by neonatal ventral hippocampal lesions in rats. Neuropsychopharmacology 2006;31:1382–92.

Index

Posttest

To receive your certificate of CME credit or participation, please complete the posttest (you must score at least 70% to receive credit) and activity evaluation answer sheet found on the last page and return it by mail or fax it to (1)-760-931-8713. Once received, your posttest will be graded and, along with your certificate (if a score of 70% or more was attained), returned to you by mail. Alternatively, you may complete these items online and immediately print your certificate at **www.neiglobal.com/pt/08minibook1**. There is a $30 fee for CME credits for this activity (waived for NEI members).

Please circle the correct answer on the answer sheet provided.

1. Dopamine in schizophrenia is hypothetically:
   A. hyperactive in the mesolimbic and ni-grostriatal pathways, and hypoactive in the mesocortical pathway
   B. hypoactive in the mesolimbic pathway, and of normal activity in the mesocortical and nigrostriatal pathways
   C. hyperactive in the mesolimbic pathway, hypoactive in the mesocortical pathway, and of normal activity in the nigrostriatal pathway
   D. hypoactive in the mesolimbic and mesocortical pathways, and hyperactive in the nigrostriatal pathway

2. Serotonin 2A receptors:
   A. lead to decreased dopamine release when stimulated
   B. are located on GABA interneurons and on somatodendritic and axonal regions of dopamine receptors
   C. act as dopamine accelerators, thus increasing dopamine release when stimulated
   D. A and B
   E. B and C
   F. A and C

3. As opposed to dopamine release, glutamate release is
   A. increased by stimulation of 5HT2A receptors
   B. increased by stimulation of 5HT1A receptors
   C. decreased by stimulation of 5HT2A receptors
   D. unaffected by serotonin receptors

4. Chronic D2 receptor blockade:

A. leads to receptor downregulation

C. prevents the occurrence of tardive dyskinesia

B. induces an increase in prolactin levels

D. does not happen with conventional D2 antipsychotics

5. Extrapyramidal side effects are more prominent in antipsychotics with:

A. rapid D2 dissociation

C. D2 partial agonist actions

B. 5HT2A antagonist properties

D. tight binding to D2 receptors

For questions 6-8, match the symptoms to the receptor:
With regard to conventional antipsychotics, which side effect is linked to which receptor blockade?

6. weight gain

A. alpha 1 receptor

7. constipation

B. histamine 1 receptor

8. low blood pressure

C. muscarinic 1 receptor

9. Various antipsychotics have been effective at treating mood and cognitive disorders due to their actions at which receptors?

A. alpha 2, histamine1, and norepi-nephrine transporter

C. Alpha 2, 5HT1A/2C, and norepi-nephrine transporter

B. Muscarinic 1, dopamine 2, and 5HT1A/2C

10. Injectable formulations of some antipsychotics can be used in an emergency case to treat which of the following symptoms?

A. negative

D. cognitive

G. B and C

B. positive

E. A and B

H. B and D

C. aggressive

F. A and C

I. all of the above

11. Cigarette smoking can impact the metabolism of which antipsychotics? Those metabolized by the:

A. CYP450 2D6 enzymes

C. CYP450 3A4 enzymes

B. CYP450 1A2 enzymes

D. CYP450 2C9 enzymes

12. A recommended strategy for using a benzodiazepine in a patient with schizophrenia is when:

A. switching between sedating antipsy-chotics

C. switching from a sedating to a nonse-dating antipsychotic

B. one is trapped in cross-titration of antipsychotic

D. everything else fails

13. Which receptors are involved in sedation?

A. D2, 5HT2A, H1 and alpha2

C. D2, M1, H1 and alpha1

B. M1, H1 and 5HT2C

D. D1, 5HT3, M3 and alpha2

14. Which two antipsychotics to date have the lowest cardiometabolic and weight gain risk?

A. clozapine and olanzapine

C. risperidone and quetiapine

B. aripiprazole and ziprasidone

D. ziprasidone and clozapine

Stahl's Neuroscience and Mental Health Pocketbook Series: Antipsychotics
Posttest and Activity Evaluation Answer Sheet

Please complete the posttest and activity evaluation answer sheet on this page and return by mail or fax. Alternatively, you may complete these items online and immediately print your certificate at **www.neiglobal.com/pt/08minibook1**. (Circle the correct answer)

Posttest Answer Sheet (score of 70% or higher required for CME credit)

1.	A B C D	8.	A B C
2.	A B C D E F	9.	A B C
3.	A B C D	10.	A B C D E F G H I
4.	A B C D	11.	A B C D
5.	A B C D	12.	A B C D
6.	A B C	13.	A B C D
7.	A B C	14.	A B C D

Activity Evaluation: Please rate the following, using a scale of:

    1-poor   2-below average   3-average   4-above average   5-excellent

1. The overall quality of the content   1   2   3   4   5

2. The relevance of the content to my professional needs   1   2   3   4   5

3. The level at which the learning objective was met of teaching me to describe the hypothetical neurobiology of schizophrenia   1   2   3   4   5

4. The level at which the learning objective was met of teaching me to understand the complex pharmacology of antipsychotics   1   2   3   4   5

5. The level at which the learning objective was met of teaching me to recognize how different drug properties affect the various symptoms of schizophrenia   1   2   3   4   5

6. The level at which the learning objective was met of teaching me to recognize that side effects are linked to the drug's receptor profile   1   2   3   4   5

7. The level at which the learning objective was met of teaching me to develop an understanding of the best treatment practices and switching methods for schizophrenia   1   2   3   4   5

8. The level at which this activity was objective, scientifically balanced, and free of commercial bias   1   2   3   4   5

9. The overall quality of this activity
(continued on next page)   1   2   3   4   5

10. Based on my experience and knowledge, the level of this activity was:

        Too Basic   Basic   Appropriate   Complex   Too Complex

11. Based on the information presented in this activity, I will:

    A.   Change my practice
    B.   Seek additional information on this topic
    C.   Do nothing as current practice reflects activity's recommendations
    D.   Do nothing as the content was not convincing

12. What barriers might keep you from implementing changes in your practice you'd like to make as a result of participating in this activity?

13. The following additional information about this topic would help me in my practice:

14. How could this activity have been improved?

15. Additional comments:

Name: _____ Credentials: _____

Address: _____

City, State, Zip: _____

Email: _____ Phone: _____

Method of Payment: Check   Visa   Mastercard   NEI Member # _____

Credit Card #: _____ Exp. Date: _____

Signature: _____ Date: _____

Amount Authorized: $30.00

Mail or fax both sides of this form to:

CME Department
Neuroscience Education Institute
1930 Palomar Point Way, Suite 101
Carlsbad, CA 92008
Fax: 760-931-8713